PATIENTS AND THEIR DOCTORS
The Journey through Medical Care

For
James, Catherine, Patrick
and Julia

PATIENTS AND THEIR DOCTORS

The Journey through Medical Care

GLIN BENNET

MA, MD, FRCS, MRCPsych

Department of Mental Health, University of Bristol

BAILLIÈRE TINDALL · LONDON

A BAILLIÈRE TINDALL book published by
Cassell Ltd,
35 Red Lion Square, London WC1R 4SG

and at Sydney, Auckland, Toronto, Johannesburg

an affiliate of
Macmillan Publishing Co. Inc.
New York

First published 1979

ISBN 0 7020 0745 5

Typeset by Scribe Design, Medway, Kent
Printed in Great Britain by Billings and Sons Ltd,
Guildford and Worcester

British Library Cataloguing in Publication Data

Bennet, Glin
 Patients and their doctors.
 1. Hospital patients — Psychology
 2. Physicians — Psychology
 I. Title
 363.1 ' 1   RC965.3

ISBN 0-7020-0745-5

Contents

Preface

Illness provides doctors with their livelihood, identity and opportunities for distinction: illness causes patients to suffer. Doctors need patients just as patients need doctors. The relationship between them is intimate because they are both involved in their very different ways with the illness itself.

This book is about the experience of sick people, because illness has a meaning and significance beyond the descriptions of pathology. It is also about the experience of doctors, since the actual business of treating ill people is seldom the doctor's prime preoccupation. Doctors and patients each have their special needs, and how these blend or collide inevitably has a bearing on the quality of health care.

To develop these themes the book is divided into three sections which emphasize different aspects: the illness, patients, and doctors. First of all, Chapters 1 and 2 deal with illnesses, and ways of looking at them not normally employed by doctors. Next, chapters 3 to 10 are mainly about patients, starting with the patient's first encounter with the doctor, then following his or her journey through the medical machine — entering hospital, awaiting surgery, postoperative and intensive care, experiencing pain, disability and finally dying.

Doctors are the subject of the last four chapters. The importance of what doctors do gives them enormous power and most of the time they act in a way which increases their dominance and emphasizes the helplessness of patients. In their private lives, however, doctors present a sorry picture,

with high rates for suicide, divorce, alcoholism, drug abuse
and psychiatric consultation; all of which contrast sharply
with their outward appearances of success. They have
prejudices and idiosyncracies like everyone else, but their
great power allows these to be acted out unchecked. In the
last chapter, The Wounded Physician, an outline is given of
the kind of doctor who practices medicine, not from a
position of apparent omnipotence and infallibility, but as a
human being who acknowledges that he is potentially as
vulnerable as anyone else in society and who can allow the
patient to participate in the process of healing.

Although primarily addressed to doctors and medical
students, with the object of trying to make them more aware
of what they are doing in their daily round and of how their
various interventions are perceived by their patients, the
book is intended for all those who have any dealing with the
sick and want to study illness in a broader context.

It is also something of a personal book arising from my
having worked before taking up psychiatry in most kinds of
medical establishment, and from my having carried out most
kinds of medical treatment and performed practically all the
standard sugrical operations. I mention this because when
writing about general hospitals and what goes on in them I
am inevitably looking back at many of the regrettable things
I have done in the past or suspect that I may have done, and
writing, therefore, with the humility and licence of an
intimate and participant, not as a judgemental outsider.

The examples used are inevitably selective, and the story is
set in hospital, but the examples illustrate general themes
which I believe apply widely. Doctors will react to the
section on doctors in their own way. As a doctor myself, I
cannot pretend to be objective, but the issues in that section
concern aspects of a doctor's life which seem to me to be
important, and with which I have tried to grapple myself.

I hope also that this book will be useful as a work of
reference, as there is much valuable writing about illness
which appears in publications not normally seen by doctors.
For reasons of space and readability a great deal which could
have been said has been left out but I have tried to
compensate for this by being generous with references. There

are fashions in research, with the result that a cluster of studies is made in a short space of time and then nothing more is heard, so some of the sources cited may strike the reader as old, but they can still be disturbingly relevant as with some of the studies of communication in hospitals (Chapter 4). I have used the pronoun 'he' quite often when referring to either sex because repeatedly to write 'he or she' seemed to me to be cumbersome, but I hope I shall not have offended any readers.

Finally, I am deeply grateful to the many patients whose experiences have illustrated themes in this book, and to my medical and surgical colleagues in various specialties. In particular I would like to thank Professor D. Russell Davis for much valuable advance, Jacqueline Barton for her help with the overall design as well as for her detailed criticism and editing of the final text, Nadia Duggan who prepared the entire manuscript, and Linda Bennet who created the setting for the work and provided constant encouragement.

GLIN BENNET

January 1979

1. Meaning in Illness

The great success of Western medicine has been in finding answers to the question 'How?': discovering *how* illness is transmitted, *how* it becomes established in the body, and *how* it can be cured or relieved. It all adds up to an immense achievement, and the success story continues as institutions and professions flourish. The advances nowadays are spectacular. They dazzle doctors and the general public alike until we scarcely notice that something vitally important has been lost along the way.

There is more to illness than a sequence of purely physical processes. Everyone would agree with that, but medicine has come to be dominated by technology, and the concepts and language of technology are only suited to describing physical events.

In the past when someone fell ill people asked 'Why?'. Why that person? Why at that time? What had the person done to bring down such misfortune? This kind of thinking was natural in many early communities where there was a sense of relatedness to the environment, which comprised not only other people but animals, plants, the physical surroundings and the seasonal and planetary cycles. It was expected that a disturbance in one part of the system would inevitably be felt throughout the whole. Within the individual also there was a sense of unity, and no separation of psychological and physical events.

Within this system the appearance of illness was likely to be taken to mean that the individual had somehow got out of

1

equilibrium with himself and his environment. Such an approach to illness provided a meaning which enabled people to cope with sufferings which could not be relieved. With a few conspicuous exceptions this view of illness prevailed in the world until the time of the enlightenment in Europe in the seventeenth century.

Around this time two basic ideas were gaining wide currency in Europe. They were to lead to radically new ways of thinking about illness and, more importantly, to new initiatives in the relief of physical suffering. First was the idea that the world functioned according to rational laws which were open to human understanding. Thus disease could be seen as a natural rather than a supernatural phenomenon (this, of course, was the view of the Hippocratic school twenty centuries earlier but their teachings had been disregarded for most of this time).

Secondly, the philosophical splitting of the mind from the body provided an intellectual framework in which the observer could stand back and be separate from the object of his study. In medicine this has led to a massive accumulation of information about the structure and function of the body and about the processes of disease.

Medicine allied itself with the physical sciences, and many of the assumptions were shared. The body, after all, was a mechanism, although a very complicated one. A great many bodily functions — circulation of the blood, filtration in the kidneys, electrical conduction along nerve fibres — were known to operate in accordance with the principles of physical science, and there was no reason to suppose that the same should not apply to all bodily (and psychological) processes.

In the realm of diseases the mechanistic view was widely demonstrated. The processes of diabetes mellitus, worked out in the 1920s, provide a typical example. Steroids, prostaglandins and other agents reveal fascinating mechanisms within the body, which can sometimes lead to dramatic therapeutic advances. Mental disorder also has been associated with demonstrable physical processes, as in the case of phenylketonuria. No doubt there are many more subtle and beautiful mechanisms yet to be discovered.

Such processes are fascinating but they are answering the question 'How?' and not 'Why?'. It is natural for the scientist to investigate how things happen. Indeed *what* happens and *how* it happens have been the dominating themes of scientific investigation over the last three hundred years, so much so that it is hard for the Westerner to imagine how he would begin investigating anything unless such questions were framed at the outset. In medicine this approach has been so successful and has attracted so much prestige to the medical profession that there has been little incentive or pressure to question the fundamental assumptions.

More than a century ago physicists made observations which could not be explained within the existing theories. Doubtless some of the workers denied the validity of such observations, but there were some, like Max Planck[1], who realized that new models of explanation were needed, and in time totally new ideas were elaborated such as relativity theory and quantum theory. Physicists were liberated by these discoveries in the sense that they became able to approach questions of empirical observation and causality in a much more realistic way. Physicists also learned how to live with uncertainty without losing their intellectual rigour.

Unfortunately, medical science, from the conceptual (though not from the technological) point of view, has remained stuck somewhere in the middle of the nineteenth century. Doctors want to be regarded as 'scientific' but they tend to restrict themselves to physical processes which can be observed directly and measured numerically. Social and psychological processes cannot be quantified numerically most of the time, and they tend to be disregarded[2]. Thus much that is recordable is lost.

The technology of medicine has run way ahead of thinking about the nature of and meaning of illness. 'Why has this man fallen ill?' is a question that is simply never asked in Western society. Yet the question is relevant. It is important to know why this man fell ill, why he fell ill when he did, and why it was he and not his twin brother. Serious illness or a surgical operation can alter the whole course of a person's life. The factors which determine a happy or a fatal outcome are complex, and they extend far beyond considerations of pathological processes. The person's conceptualizations about the nature of disease, his previous experience of it, his state of mind and the social environment in its broadest sense, all feed into the problem. A proper understanding of a person's illness requires consideration of all these factors, and it requires a way of thinking about illness which can accommodate a vast amount of assorted information.

A balance of health and disease

In the late 1960s when computers were beginning to appear on the clinical scene, questions of definition attracted the attention of medical theoreticians[3,4] on the grounds that if terms such as 'disease' and 'health' and 'normality' were going to be used in connection with computers, the terms ought in principle to be defined. Even now, to my knowledge, no writer has produced a definition of any of these terms which even he himself regards as satisfactory. Apart from anything else, the borderland between health and disease is an endless grey area because of the number of variables involved. If one measure, such as blood pressure, is involved, it is hard to say even for a given individual at what point it becomes pathological. If more than one variable is involved — as will always be the case in practice — the cut-off point between health and disease becomes completely indefinable.[5]

Perhaps difficulties in definition have arisen because the wrong questions are being asked, and these may follow from certain assumptions people hold about the nature of health and disease — in particular, disease and health as discrete entities. In day-to-day practice it is perfectly reasonable to say that, 'this person is healthy', or 'that person is ill', and such assertions may lead to useful action. When we try to get beyond the physical processes of disease to understand something about the nature of health and disease, it becomes less satisfactory to separate the two states as though they were mutually exclusive. A man with one leg may lead a vigorous and productive life, another person with no demonstrable physical or mental disorder may be a hopeless invalid: which of these is healthy and which diseased?

Traditionally, a fully developed disease is seen as the end of a sequence of events where there are strict causal connections between each step. Where the processes of disease are concerned it is reasonable to look for such connections, and they impose a useful intellectual control on the observer. However, if a strict causal sequence is considered essential, then only those phenomena which can be fitted into a neat chain of events will be recorded, and all other information will be disregarded.

Although the processes of development of pathological states can be viewed as a causally connected sequence of events, I do not believe that the origins of illness should be. Health is a state of dynamic equilibrium in which all kinds of forces within and outside the individual are held in balance. These forces (or tendencies) comprise genetically determined factors, idiosyncracies of constitution, individual temperament and personality, mental state and physical state, every kind of life experience — especially those concerned with threat or loss — and all the occurrences — physical and psychological — in the person's environment. This amounts to an infinitely large collection of influences, and it would be impossible to set them into a causal framework. A causal approach cannot be illuminating in this area, any more than it can be in sub-atomic physics. In technology, yes, and the same goes for the practical technology of clinical medicine, but when it comes to trying to understand something about the nature and meaning of an illness a more 'organic' view has to be taken. 'Organic' here is used to denote the interrelatedness of all things and events — including the observer — and it stands in contrast to the 'mechanistic' view where causal sequences are expected and the observer stands back from the object under study.

The organic view implies a harmony or balance of forces in nature. This was exemplified in the work of some of the early Greek philosophers such as Heraclitus and Pythagoras (and in the east in the teachings of the Taoists with their conception of the *yang* and the *yin*), and it is fundamental in the Hippocratic system. It is unfortunate that these valuable ideas were thrown out along with Hippocrates' erroneous physiology at the time of the rise of empirical science.

When all forces — physical, psychological, environmental — are in balance health exists: when they are out of balance the individual may fall ill.

These ideas are described here not as a theory of disease (or perhaps one should talk about the continuum 'health–disease') but simply as a useful way of making sense of the numerous factors which affect the individual in the course of living. This book will be concerned with many of these influences and will draw on all kinds of sources. A proper understanding of illness — why people fall ill, why they fail to recover as expected — requires us to take account of as much as possible of the available information, and as doctors to learn more about the curious interrelationship of doctors and patients.

Summary

Western technological medicine has been abundantly success-ful in answering questions about *how* diseases develop. Little attention has been paid to *why* they develop, or to basic questions about the nature of health and disease. Perhaps health and disease should not be regarded as totally separate entities, and an 'organic' view is presented in which good health is seen as no more than a state of equilibrium between opposing physical, psychological and environmental forces acting upon the individual.

2. Non-medical Views of Illness

Everyone in society is a potential patient, and illness interests everyone. It has been widely studied by non-medical workers in the social sciences[1] for whom the significance of illness in society or in the individual is of more interest than the technical minutiae of pathological processes. Three such approaches will be discussed briefly in this chapter under the headings (1) sick role; (2) life events and illness; and (3) personality and susceptibility to illness.

Sick role — or being a patient

In Western society a generally kindly view is taken of the sick. Brutalities may be perpetrated upon the healthy; the 'sick' will be left in peace. Talcott Parsons,[2] an American sociologist, has identified what he calls the 'sick role' to describe some of the ways illness is perceived in contemporary society, the ways people regard and behave towards the sick, and the expectations society has of those it has chosen to define as sick.

1. The sick are relieved from the normal social responsibilites, in particular working and earning a living. On the other hand anyone who claims such exemptions without 'really' being sick will be judged to be malingering and will be punished by society.

2. The sick are not held responsible for their incapacity, and it will be assumed that they will need to be looked after.

Those who poison themselves with drugs and alcohol, however, are seen as responsible for their actions and so are often treated harshly by the caring professions.

3. Sickness is regarded as a misfortune, and so it is assumed that the sick will want to get well. The hypochondriac, or any person who seems to delight in the possession of symptoms, does not behave as though sickness is a misfortune and so will not be received kindly by doctors or by society in general.

4. The sick are obliged to seek competent medical help, and to do all they can to get well. The neurotic person can be rejected because he (or she) can appear unwilling to take constructive steps towards overcoming the disabling symptoms.

The concept of the sick role immediately takes illness beyond considerations of pathological processes, of signs and symptoms and diagnostic categories. It becomes part of the broader relationship an individual has with society. Although the concept is enunciated in terms of effects of illness, these effects or consequences may be attractive in their own right and may have a substantial part to play in the origins of illness or the failure to recover as expected — provided of course that the sufferers obey all the rules of the person in the sick role. Doctors should not feel that they are somehow outside this system. If anything, doctors interpret the sick role conditions (in terms of what is expected of patients) more rigidly than any others in society, and I think the ones who interpret it most rigidly are the ones who would least like to acknowledge their debt to a sociologist.

Life events and illness

Before the Age of Enlightenment there was no difficulty in accepting that how someone felt could have a bearing on how that person lived, or in some cases on how that person came to die. Sir Henry Wootton (1598–1639) wrote this tender couplet 'Upon the death of Sir Albert Morton's wife'

> He first deceased; she for a little tried
> To live without him, liked it not, and died.

Even as late as the middle of the seventeenth century 'Griefe' was listed as a cause of death in Heberden's mortality tables for London,[3] but it has taken doctors three hundred years to work though the implications of the philosophy of the Enlightenment so that they can once again recognize that the experiences a person has in life really can have an effect on health. Even so, I doubt if this recognition would have occurred if the associations between life events and illness had not been presented with contemporary epidemiological and statistical precision.

There is now a large literature on bereavement, and it is well known that morbidity and mortality rates among the recently bereaved are likely to be high.[3] It is less widely appreciated that other kinds of loss are also associated with poor health,[4-7] and I had a chance to study this prospectively when some 3000 houses in Bristol were flooded in 1968.[8]

In a sample of the flooded population I found that attendances at general practioners' surgeries increased by 53% in the year following the flooding, and referrals to hospital outpatient departments and hospital admissions more than doubled (as compared with a control group which had not been flooded). The reasons for hospital admission did not suggest any direct consequences of exposure and were a more or less random series of diagnoses. The overall mortality rate in the flooded area increased by 50%, with the most pronounced rise in the age group 45 to 64. Of special (but unexplained) interest here were the deaths from malignant disease. In the year before the flooding there were nine deaths, during the year after there were 21, with negligible change for the rest of Bristol. Similar results were found on examination of the mortality rates following the severe flooding of Canvey Island in the Thames estuary,[9] after inundation from the sea in 1953.

A detailed investigation into the health of a diverse population of New Yorkers over a twenty-year period showed that not only does illness 'cluster' at certain periods in a person's life (one-third of a person's illnesses occurred in one-eighth of the time) but that it is by no means randomly distributed throughout the population. Thus, one-quarter of the study population had one-half the illnesses, while the quarter at the other end of the scale had less than one tenth of them. L.E. Hinkle and Harold Wolff,[10] both important contributors to knowledge about the social antecedents to illness, concluded that 'the great majority of clusters of illness episodes . . . occurred at times when [people] perceived their life situations to be unsatisfying, threatening, overdemanding, and productive of conflict, and they could make no satisfactory adaptation to these situations. The situations were, in general, those which arose out of disturbed relations with family members and important associates, threats to security and status, and restrictions . . . which made it impossible to satisfy important needs and drives.'

The key remark is '. . . they could make no satisfactory adaptation to these situations'. And then emphasizing 'family members and important associates . . .' In other words, it is most of all the experience of *frustration* − especially where personal relationships are involved − that generates the tensions that lead to symptoms.

For many people the association between a distressing experience in life and subsequent illness is obvious, and there is no need for statistical 'proof'. However, researchers always want to refine their methods, and in this area of study it has led to attempts at quantification of life events. This approach has been pressed to the furthest degree by Rahe and his associates in San Diego and elsewhere[11,12] who have evolved a scoring system in which events could be assigned a numerical value to indicate their relative importance as psychosocial antecedents of illness. This simple numerical approach to illness does have some value as a research tool but it can be criticised on technical grounds.[13-15] I find it unsatisfying in general because it takes no account of the individual's experience of the event, his feelings about it and its unique meaning for him at the particular time the event (or events) occurred. However, in clinical practice, an enquiry about recent life events is always easy to make, and it is often illuminating when symptoms are found to date from a distressing experience, or an ongoing social problem is discovered which suddenly makes sense of a patient's failure to recover as expected.

Personality and susceptibility to illness

The events in a person's life have some relationship to the incidence of illness, but what about the sufferer himself? Are there personal attributes which play a part in the development of illness, either by rendering someone more susceptible to illnesses in general or else by endowing him with a specific vulnerability in an organ or system of the body?[16,17]

These personal aspects can be said to comprise the personality, by which I mean certain enduring patterns of behaviour irrespective of whether these are genetically determined or the result of experiences in early childhood.

Coronary artery disease and personality

Here is a pattern of behaviour which most doctors can recognize in themselves, and also among their patients and their colleagues. It is called Type A behaviour by the two San Francisco physicians, Meyer Friedman and Ray H. Rosenman, who described it.[18-20]

The Type A man has:
1. An intense, sustained drive to achieve self-selected but usually poorly defined goals.
2. A continuous involvement in multiple activities which are liable to be subjected to real or imaginary deadlines.
3. A habit of accentuating explosively various key words in ordinary speech, and of hurrying the ends of sentences.
4. A persistent desire to compete and to receive recognition, and aggressive tendencies towards others of similar temperament.
5. Brisk body movements, fist clenching, rapid eating, great difficulty in relaxing and guilty feelings when not engaged in any specific activity.
6. Great physical and mental alertness but little 'time to spare to become the things worth *being* because of the preoccupation with getting the things worth *having*'.

By contrast, among those described as exhibiting Type B behaviour, 'the most striking difference was the relative or complete absence of the sense of time urgency . . . Most men of group B were obviously more content with their respective lot in life and relatively uninterested in pursuing multiple goals or competitive activities.'

Type A behaviour is associated with coronary artery disease, as are also parental coronary artery disease, cigarette smoking, and raised serum cholesterol and raised diastolic blood pressure. Friedman and Rosenman say that Type A behaviour is the most important correlate. Severe coronary atherosclerosis was found to be around twice as common among Type A individuals dying from any cause than among Type Bs also dying from any cause.[21] Conversely, a Type B man was regarded as being virtually immune from coronary artery disease if his serum cholesterol and triglycerides were in the low normal range.

For many people the formulation of the Type A and Type B behaviour patterns immediately rings true, painfully so among those who are reappraising their life-style after a recent myocardial infarct. Others complain that the association has not been 'proved', in the same way that the association between smoking and lung cancer has not been 'proved'. To demand outright proof from any investigation involving human behaviour seems to me to indicate a failure to grasp the complexity of human beings when they are studied as a whole. Friedman and Rosenman's theory *a priori feels* authentic, and almost twenty years of subsequent research has failed to unseat it.[22,23] It is, of course, not the first time such ideas have been advanced. In 1897 Sir William Osler[24] pointed out how the most worthy and hard working citizens were the ones most prone to myocardial infarction, and Flanders Dunbar[25,26] in the 1930s and 1940s made extensive observations of patients with a variety of physical conditions and delineated a personality profile for myocardial infarction very similar to that of Friedman and Rosenman.

Personality factors in other conditions

Most of the early work on psychosomatic correlations involved a search for personality traits which were specific for particular physical conditions. Certain workers have claimed to be able to differentiate such conditions as bronchial asthma, neurodermatitis, rheumatoid arthritis, hypertension, ulcerative colitis, thyrotoxicosis, and peptic ulcer with a fair degree of reliability on the basis of psycho-social data alone[27] and others have claimed to be able to identify specific personality factors in an even broader range of diseases.[28] For many of these conditions plausible explanations have been offered in terms of maladaptive autonomic responses,[29] since most of the conventional 'psychosomatic' diseases involve physical changes which are mediated by known autonomic processes.

When it comes to personality factors in cancer the issues become much more complex because cancer is so diverse in its manifestations and the mechanisms are not understood anyway. Nevertheless, there is a large and somewhat per-plexing literature on the subject[30,31] and some workers have made a convincing case by identifying specific attitudes (mainly feelings of hopelessness about life and living) on a prospective basis.[32]

Summary

This chapter has touched upon three non-clinicopathological ways of looking at illness: the social consequences (and especially benefits) of being ill, the events in life which can increase the likelihood of falling ill, and the kind of person-ality which is particularly at risk. Often, all three factors can be taken into account with advantage, but the main point of the chapter has been to emphasize that there are ways other than the strictly medical of looking at illness, and that the doctor can improve the quality of his appraisal by taking account of information outside the traditional clinico-pathological framework.

PATIENTS, AND THE JOURNEY THROUGH MEDICAL CARE

3. Meeting the Patient

If ever I need to remind myself what a patient feels like coming to a hospital out-patient department, all I have to do is to take a five-minute walk down the hill from the Bristol Royal Infirmary to the Law Courts. I ordinarily inhabit a hospital environment where I have a distinct role and status, where the organization is totally familiar, where the uniforms and grades of staff are readily identifiable, and where no harm is likely to come to me. In court I have a function, to give evidence say, but I am not part of the organization, and certainly have no status there. It is impossible to know the details of what is going on yet there is always a sense or urgency with small groups talking earnestly in the corridors, and an outsider is unable to differentiate the figures in dark suits, black gowns, wigs and the like. The assembly of unidentifiable figures engaged in urgent but unintelligible business leaves me with an uncanny feeling that only trouble can result from the proceedings. At all costs I must not put a foot wrong or else the incomprehensible machine will somehow land me in the dock instead of the witness box.

These are the feelings that all too many patients have on entering a hospital. However, the patient's story begins not on first catching sight of the doctor but in that private moment of realization — feeling a lump in the breast, a crippling dart of pain in the back, red blood in the urine, a nagging ache which has gone on too long — that something serious has happened which is beyond the individual's resources to cope with. The experience of something being

17

wrong is then intensified by the person's imagination and previous experiences, dimly remembered newspaper articles or second-hand accounts of people with similar complaints. Thus patients may arrive at the doctor's with not only their own experiences but the garbled experience of others as well.

Consultation in hospital

First, the hospital system itself must be penetrated, and that is quite an ordeal. The older the patient, the more likely is the outcome to be serious: the newer, bigger and better equipped the hospital, the more likely it is to be impersonal. The hospital may be associated with the joy of childbirth or with the death of a close relative. Always there will be uncertainty. 'Hospitals are institutions cradled in anxiety', as one observer[1] has put it.

Doctors ordain the atmosphere of their clinics. They control the numbers and the time-tabling, so that a stroller through an out-patient department during a working afternoon may see hectic waiting areas jammed with adults and children, with distracted clinic staff bustling back and forth, or else clinics with only a few people at any one time waiting quietly for their turn with the doctor.

Inside the consultation rooms the bustling, ebullient clinician positions himself in the centre of a large room with examination cubicles leading off it. On the large desk there are piles of case notes and X-rays, and other paraphernalia. There are nurses in attendance, students also if it is a teaching hospital. The patient is shown in and sits across the desk from the consultant or else at one side of it; in either event some of the paraphernalia intervenes between doctor and patient.[2] Picture that patient's position. Anxiously he approaches the specialist. He has prepared himself for this moment just as the doctor would prepare himself for giving evidence in court. He must try to be concise, not to waste anybody's time. Everyone is busy here so he must come to the point quickly. The doctor has the nurses scurrying to and fro, he ticks off the clinic helper about a missing pathology report, answers the telephone, sifts through a pile of papers, and ever so discreetly looks at the clock. He does not need to say he is busy; indeed he may say exactly the opposite. Unwittingly he is creating an atmosphere of haste which has an inhibiting effect on all but the most insensitive of patients and can lead to a complex clinical and social problem being oversimplified to a misleading degree because the patient is unable to express the details of the problem and, most important, his feelings about it.

I suspect that what can make a long clinic so tiring physically and emotionally for the doctor is not so much seeing all those people with symptoms, but questioning and examining them without ever getting into personal contact with any one of them. Some doctors even seem to dislike patients, which is sad. I used to see something of a man regarded as the greatest clinical neurologist of his day and he did not speak to his patients 'on principle': he saw himself as providing a service to the general practitioner, that was all.

First encounter

A great deal happens before even a word is said. In the interval between the patient's catching sight of the doctor and beginning to talk, the atmosphere of the interview is established. This applies to any interpersonal encounter, but the high emotional tension that surrounds a medical consultation means that the patient will be extra sensitive to every nuance of the doctor's behaviour.[3,4] The doctor wants to be welcoming but a bone-crushing handshake and a smile with jaw jutting and teeth flashing is distinctly aggressive, and the impression is augmented by smart clothes and a commanding style of speech. The patient has either to submit or to oppose, and the good doctor wants neither of these responses. On the other hand the doctor may not even look up from his desk. In interactional terms he is being submissive, seated with his head hung and avoiding eye contact. He may also be protected behind a desk so he offers an ambiguous message — a submissive doctor but one who is also defending himself.

The encounter should be pitched somewhere between these extremes. Some simple self-help type techniques may not be out of place when we are tired and harrassed: smile deliberately at the door before the patient enters. It will make you look up from the desk and get the lines of tension off your forehead. Shake hands: it introduces a physical contact which on the whole is helpful. Some doctors recoil from it — why? Look the patient in the eye. There is nothing like concentrating on eye contact for keeping oneself riveted to the patient while inwardly tired and preoccupied.

Learn to relax. That is a subject in itself, but it is quite simple to learn to avoid complicated leg-crossing postures with an arm hung over the back of the chair. Sit with both feet squarely planted on the ground. Watch your shoulder muscles. When tense they are likely to rise up, so if the shoulders (and the jaw too) can hang loosely the chances are that the rest of the body will relax too. Every doctor should at some time take some instructions in relaxation techniques — to pass on to his patients and to use himself. Slow, deep diaphragmatic breathing, as used in *yoga,* with rapid sighing expiration, is another simple way of draining muscular tension out of the body.

Our mode of dress communicates a great deal. The expensively suited, coiffeured and manicured teaching hospital consultant is disappearing from the scene, and possibly will be replaced by the flamboyant *avant garde* type. Each is in danger of placing distance between himself and the patient. However, our style of dress is so much an expression of our personalities that we may be blind to its impact. The main thing is to be ourselves, wear what we feel good in, and not allow ourselves to conform to our fantasies of the style of our 'ideal' doctor.

Prejudice and stereotypes

Throughout the early stages of the encounter with a new patient the doctor has to make great efforts not to make prejudgements about the person before him, or assumptions about the nature of the underlying complaint. It is inevitable with common conditions such as acute appendicitis or rheumatoid arthritis, to see the syndrome as a whole, and on the basis of a few observations to make generally accurate predictions about the rest. This is a normal way of working for experienced clinicians but it can catch out the unwary if done with people as opposed to diseased parts of them.

Everyone possesses this tendency, and it is called stereotyped thinking. On the basis of a few observed phenomena, assumptions are made about other aspects of the individual's behaviour and attitudes. Obviously the process of using what is known to make inferences about what cannot be directly observed is reasonable, but where people are concerned, emotions, prejudices and moral attitudes can interfere with the process and lead to peculiar conclusions. A common contemporary stereotype involves the youth with long hair and beard, gold-rimmed spectacles, casual clothes and sandals. Without any personal contact certain members of society are prone to assume that this person is lazy, dishonest, irresponsible, unwashed, sexually promiscuous, and probably using drugs.

Stereotyped thinking can sometimes show itself in clinical medicine by the doctor recording favourable statements about the patient when he resembles the doctor in social class and attitudes, and *vice versa*. 'Intelligent, cooperative patient' generally means no more than 'middle-class'. Unfortunately there can be an element of moral censure in these stereotyped attitudes which is the main reason why it is important to recognize them.[5]

Doctors have therefore to find ways of becoming conscious of their prejudices so that they do not lapse (especially as they get older) into the trap of stereotyped thinking. Favoured areas for such thinking are the younger generation, drug usage, homosexuality, abortion, extreme left-wing political movements, apparently lenient punishments enacted by the courts and permissive sexual behaviour in general. This is not to say that anyone opposing these styles is excessively authoritarian or is necessarily indulging in stereotyped thinking; it is only so when such assumptions are made about individuals or groups of whom the critic has no direct knowledge.

A good way for anyone wondering whether or not they have a tendency to such attitudes is to discuss these and other similar topics with someone in late teenage or early twenties. Of course the very idea of discussing such matters with young people may cause embarrassment, but these same young people may have more informed and sensitive opinions about these matters than their parents and elders.

Doctors can usefully learn to monitor their reactions. Just as lecturers learn to 'think on their feet' to judge the effectiveness of their lecture and plan the next step as they are going along, so doctors can judge the progress of an interview. Just now we are interested in how the doctor is reacting to the patient as a person and to what that person is saying. Do you feel warmly towards the patient, or resentful, or angry? Does what the patient is saying evoke strong feelings in you? Take the young unmarried woman seeking an abortion. What do you feel about her as a person? Does she remind you of your daughter? Does she attract you sexually? What emotions do you feel within (as opposed to your external professional reaction) when she reveals what she wants? Does she evoke feelings relating to all young women today? And most important of all: are your emotions proportional to the clinical problem before you? Can you handle her problem calmly and sympathetically, or are you becoming tense and angry inside even though you have in front of you a frightened woman seeking help?

In short, whenever we feel ourselves experiencing hostile emotions in a clinical setting we should look into ourselves, for almost certainly that is where the real problem lies. A personal prejudice of which we have not hitherto been conscious may have been activated, or we are being confronted with a practical situation we cannot deal with.

Doctors like to be masters of every situation, death included, and this may even be a factor in the selection of medicine as a career. So doctors may be more vulnerable than most others in society to the negative emotions that can appear when they are shown to be powerless, when confronted either with an illness they cannot cure or, more commonly, with complicated psychosocial problems for which no simple solution is possible. Doctors need to recognize these negative feelings for what they are and not to react as though they were being held up as incompetents before their patients and colleagues.

Open-ended interview

The first moments of the interview are crucial. It is in these moments that the good atmosphere created by the doctor can be put to practical use. The patient has a problem, and is also anxious and receptive. There may be a medical 'complaint' but that may be no more than a ticket of entry to a medical consultation; and all too often it is far removed from the essential problem.

If the doctor opens with the question 'What are you complaining of?', he will be given a medical 'complaint' as a reply. It may be a perfectly real one and it may be the whole of the story, but since about one-third of all general practitioner consultations in England and Wales are primarily for emotional problems it clearly cannot be the whole of the story all the time.

Unfortunately, asking questions is not the best way to reach the essence of most people's problems. It puts people on the defensive, and, as Michael Balint[6] has said: 'He who asks questions will get answers, but not much else'. And even if it was the best approach no doctor could ever possibly ask enough questions to cover all eventualities, so he must foster the relaxed, accepting attitude and allow the patient to lead him to the central problem.

Such is the pressure that every patient feels consulting a doctor, especially in hospital, that the merest facilitation is often enough. Statements are better than questions, and the less directive the better. A generously delivered: 'Well now' may be enough. Or even something platitudinous like 'I've had your doctor's letter', or 'You seem to have been having some trouble'. Each doctor must work out his own style: the object of these openings is to give the patient an opportunity to indicate what is most on his mind. Surprisingly often it is some personal matter, not the presenting medical symptom, but it might be an important factor which could influence a surgeon's decision about the timing of an operation. Whatever it is it will be something worth hearing and it will establish a rapport between doctor and patient which will be helpful and satisfying to both throughout their association. And this process takes only 30 seconds or so to initiate.

It can be a revelation to doctors, once they have learned to break the habit of always having to appear to be in a hurry, and can relax long enough to allow their natural empathy to emerge, just how readily their patients (and their personal friends too no doubt) will respond to it. There may, of course, be floods of distress but along with them an even greater sense of relief and gratitude at being able, possibly for the first time ever, to express openly what really was their main concern. After that the necessary detailed questioning proceeds easily because the rapport has been established.

Influencing the patient's story

To anyone with moderate clinical experience, the patient only needs to make a few utterances concerning symptoms before the likely physical basis of the complaint becomes apparent. Indeed the very mention of 'indigestion' may have the doctor on the track of a duodenal ulcer, and thereafter he can quite unwittingly organize the patient's story to fulfil his expectations. The doctor can listen sympathetically but an observer sitting in the room might notice that the doctor shows more interest in some parts of the story than in others. The doctor's interest is manifested by his sitting up more alertly, making more eye contact, smiling, and generally relating better. During other parts of the story he sits back, his gaze wanders, he fiddles with objects on his desk. Without either party realizing it, the patient is being conditioned. Certain details the patient offers are 'rewarded' by the doctor's interest — and most patients want to please their doctor. Other items (such as psychosocial information) may be 'inhibited' by his lack of interest.

Some of the processes of diagnosis have been studied by Michael Balint[7] in his general practitioner groups in which he explored many aspects of the doctor–patient interaction, and demonstrated to what a great extent doctors control what they let patients tell them, and how selectively they hear what the patients do manage to say.

A patient relating his symptoms is making what Balint[6] calls 'offers', and the doctor replies with 'responses'. These offers contain more than simple accounts of symptoms. For example, a woman of 32 was referred who had undergone over the past three years appendicectomy, hysterectomy and cholecystectomy but was still vomiting frequently and having epigastric and retrosternal pain. Investigations revealed no abnormality. Her husband had been off work for four years, and the patient had to work full-time to support her four children. She seemed to the doctors to be an intelligent and capable woman. The patient was offering the doctors the story of someone being stretched beyond her limit, but hitherto only abdominal symptomatology had been taken into account. Once the psychosocial and interpersonal topics were opened up the vomiting and pains were to some extent replaced by manifest distress but she was helped to work directly on her problems, and she required no further surgery.

Explaining and reassuring

'I have reassured the patient that he has nothing to worry about'. such a common statement in specialists' reports but it seldom helps the patient. All too often the patient goes away simply feeling the problem has not been understood. By all means reassure, but only when reasonably satisfied that you have identified the essential problem. A 27-year-old man had an exhaustive medical investigation for left-sided chest pain, and was told that his heart and his chest were in good order and that he had nothing to worry about. He was not satisfied, and said: 'That's what they said about my dad until he died of a heart attack in the ambulance on the way to hospital'. When giving reassurance restrict it to what you know about. Explain what investigations have been done and how they can show to the best of anyone's knowledge that there is no demonstrable disease in the parts concerned. Then look beyond. This 27-year-old man had many personal problems, the most pressing of which was his mother's very early remarriage to a close friend of his father.

Often the specialist's suspicions are of something serious — a breast lump, for example. Optimistic remarks about 'cysts' or 'benign lumps' are unwise and unfair to the patient. They serve only to spare the specialist any embarrassment he might feel about using the word 'cancer' in his dealings with the patient, though most women will have suspected it from the start. The patient will worry even more if she feels her doctor has not recognized the possibility, that he does not realize how serious the lump might be. Therefore give the patient an opportunity at the end of the interview: 'Is there anything at all you would like to ask me'?

Having introduced a serious possible diagnosis, no one is going to complain unduly if the final diagnosis is something harmless. If the diagnosis does turn out to be serious then doctor and patient have already established a rapport of trust which can greatly assist the doctor, and can support the patient during the next stages.

Communicating information

The anxiety which surrounds all interactions in hospitals serves to impair communications between doctors and patients to a serious degree. It is one of the minor ironies of medical education that it implants in doctors an immense account of technical knowledge and expertise but practically nothing about how to deliver it for the benefit of the patient.

Just how badly doctors perform is shown in a recent review of surveys of communication[8] in which on average patients forgot almost half of what was told them. This is probably one of the reasons why around half the medicines prescribed by doctors are never consumed.[9,10] Patients have their own beliefs, attitudes and conceptual systems about illness, together with all kinds of prejudices (good and bad) about doctors. They also may be ignorant of medical terms obvious to the doctor. Only a fifth of a sample in Glasgow could locate the stomach correctly, and there was wide disagreement about the meanings of such terms as 'diarrhoea' and 'a medicine'.[11]

Anything that can be written down should be written down, and there is a definite place for properly designed printed instructions. Verbal communication can be improved by what is called 'explicit categorization'.[8] Here the doctor says to the patient 'I am going to tell you what is wrong, what the treatment will be, what tests will be necessary', and so on. Then he goes on: 'Now, first, what is wrong with you is . . . Secondly, what the treatment will be is . . . ' etc.

This chapter has been opening up for scrutiny the details of what goes on when doctor and patient come face to face. A self-consciousness of what is going on when two people meet may seem to some to inhibit a truly emphatic and spontaneous rapport but I have not found this to be the case in practice, any more than the discussion of the details of a personal relationship will necessarily weaken the spontaneity and feeling in that relationship. The benefits of self-awareness are that the doctor is going to make a more uniform and regular rapport, and that he will continue to make good contact even when harrassed or possibly feeling hostile towards patients in general.

Summary

A number of quite subtle processes are involved in the business of patient coming face to face with doctor. There is the physical arrangement of the consultation room, the doctor's own prejudices and how these can influence the interview, the importance of gesture and non-verbal communication, the vital open-ended start to every interview, how the doctor can unwittingly influence what the patient tells him and organize the patient's unstructured story into a conventional case-history. The requirements of effective explanation and reassurance, and communication of instructions are described.

4. Hospitals and their Inhabitants

If an appointment at a hospital out-patient department can be likened to an appearance in court, then admission to hospital can resemble going to prison.

Anyone sick enough to need to go into hospital is in no position to complain, and so has no effective rights. Sickness enforces recumbent passivity; the large ward, the institutional garments and the lack of personal belongings encourage anonymity. As in prison the patient has an official number and indistinctive clothing. In prison the sanctions are manifest, for every window has bars: in hospital, on the other hand, everyone professes to be working for the patient's good. But which institution generates the greater anxiety?

In the past I have enjoyed the cosiness and camaraderie that came from working long, hard hours and living in a hospital. The work seemed self-evidently worthwhile and the institution obviously good. I was proud to belong, and hurt the day after my appointment ended when I found I had immediately become an outsider. I have known workers in penal institutions who felt and spoke in the same way about *their* organizations. It seems strange to the unitiated that anyone could feel this way about hospitals and prisons but it is merely a phenomenon of all large institutions which, after they reach a certain size, become a way of life themselves and spawn all kinds of activities quite unconnected with the original objectives.

As doctors we perceive hospitals in a special way for we have emotionally grown up in them and have been moulded

by them. At first we were uncertain medical students, with
our short white coats and symbolic stethescopes, and at that
stage we were still identified with the general public and so
responded with dismay to the suffering we saw around us. We
could not make sense of all the people working in the
hospital, and everything we did in those early days seemed to
bring a reprimand. But soon we found we could associate
ourselves with the doctors in the longer white coats, and we
found if we adopted their manners and their style the organization could begin to make sense, and what is more it could
give us an advantageous role in that organization. In time we
came to realize that the hospital was the arena where we
would have to display our competence and professional
promise. If we wanted to advance our careers we would have
to convince our superiors and teachers that we were not only
able, but also the kind of person they wanted in the higher
echelons of medicine. Needless to say, this encourages the
conservative kind of person who could accept the gloomy
principle, which applies to hospitals as to all large organizations, that change can only be initiated by those who
benefit from the existing system. There were of course the
future general practitioners, the majority in fact. They would
want one job if possible at the teaching hospital but at an
early stage they were separated out as a kind of medical
proletariat from whom eccentricities could be tolerated and
so the pressures upon them were less.

The future specialists, as students or junior doctors, and
of course the established specialists themselves, used to
dominate the hospital. They still hold the control, though
slightly less easily since they have been joined by the brigade
of powerful hospital administrators, who, although they may
not leave all the power in the hands of the specialists, share
an interest in maintaining the technological bureaucracy
which the modern large hospital has become. Thus the
doctor's view of the hospital's function is only a fraction of
the story. Administrators, nurses, professional and technical
and other workers likewise have their viewpoints which
inevitably are linked to their own interests. So too it seems
does the Department of Health and Social Security, for how
else could they pay the McKinsey Corporation around

£220 000 to study the structure of the British National
Health Service without any consideration of the needs or
attitudes of the consumers — the patients.[1]

Hospitals are extraordinary organizations which lately
have grown too large, too expensive, too inflexible, too
political, and caring for the sick has ceased to be their sole
function. Indeed it would be possible to remove all the
patients from some teaching hospitals and the organization
would roll on for some time before anyone noticed. For an
intelligible sociological view of hospitals the reader is referred
to David Tuckett's *Introduction to Medical Sociology*[1] but
I prefer to study an organization in terms of the different
kinds of people involved in it, their points of view, their
problems and their relationships with other groups.

Patients

What does it mean to be a patient in a large hospital? Is it
like staying in a big hotel, where no trouble is spared to
ensure the guest's quiet enjoyment? Or like public transport,
where the traveller pays heavily for a ticket and then feels
treated with condescension? It is really very hard to say. It is
always publicly implied that the hospital organization
revolves around the patient's needs. This is clearly not what
happens, but where does the patient fit into the organization
as a whole, and what is his experience?[2,3]

For many, of course, the experience is smooth, and in
retrospect agreeable, but this may be determined to a greater
extent by the patient's personality than by the nature of the
illness itself. The patient who is cheerful, pleasant, grateful,
amusing, understanding, optimistic, interesting to nurse, and
who needs intensive nursing, is likely to be best regarded by
the nursing staff; and the relationship with the nursing staff is
the factor most likely to determine the overall experience of
hospital. On the other hand the patient who is seen as selfish,
bad-tempered, grumbling, unwilling to accept treatment,
reluctant to go home, not needing to be in hospital, who is
foreign, has a psychiatric diagnosis, or has been in hospital
more than three months, may have less good recollections.
These were some of the conclusions of a survey into nursing

attitudes published by the Royal College of Nursing and entitled *The Unpopular Patient.*[4] These expectations and attitudes are shared by all staff (except perhaps social workers), and can readily be heard whenever staff are talking about the patients. So great is the power that staff have in controlling every aspect of the patient's existence in hospital that inevitably a conditioning process operates, of which few are consciously aware, to ensure that patients behave in a way that suits the staff. Those who will not or cannot meet these expectations are always in danger of rejection.

I was asked to see a 63-year-old man in a general ward who had been admitted with retention of urine a few days previously. He had evidently been pulling his catheter out, had refused to be weighed and was accusing the staff of plotting against him. They had sedated him but without effect. When I approached him, I drew the curtains around the bed, pulled up a chair, sat down saying nothing more than a simple greeting. Almost straight away he said: 'I just don't know what they want me to do'. He went on to explain that he was trying to help the nurses with their work but did not know how to. The nursing staff for their part had come to feel that he was being deliberately uncooperative or else was mentally disturbed, and considerable antagonism had developed. It therefore seemed best to transfer him to the psychiatric unit. Whether it was the carpets, curtains and divan beds in the psychiatric unit or simply the quieter atmosphere, we shall never know, but from the moment he entered the unit he was mentally perfectly normal. It turned out that he had had a mild degree of prostatic enlargement for some time, and more recently had become mildly depressed, for which tricyclic antidepressants had been prescribed. These had quite possibly precipitated the acute retention which led to his admission to hospital in severe physical discomfort and some personal distress. Describing the events in retrospect, he said he never knew what was going on, where he was being taken to and what they were going to do to him. It is likely that the combined effect of all these factors rendered him unable to comprehend and interpret his surroundings, and so he became disorientated, and also highly anxious, which compounded the problem. A negative reaction from the staff towards this 'confused old man' merely made him worse until they really did have a problem patient on their hands. Such is the pressure upon staff in accident departments and acute surgical wards that they do not have time to explain, yet a few words early on before this man had been bracketed a 'good' or a 'difficult' patient would have prevented the whole subsequent chain of events.

What constitutes 'good' behaviour in patients is never precisely stated: it is merely that which pleases the staff. In this way general hospitals join the ranks of what Erving Goffman[5] has called 'total institutions', which comprise orphanages, old people's homes, mental hospitals, prisons, army barracks, ships, boarding schools, monasteries, convents, anywhere which provides total care for its members and demands a stern measure of conformity. These institutions vary, of course, in the outward intensity of their methods of control, but they do all aim to control totally, and they share a number of techniques for achieving this.

One of these techniques of particular interest to us has been called 'stripping'. It is the process whereby the new patient is stripped of the outward signs of individuality by the removal of clothes and personal possessions, including the various bits and pieces most people need if they are to look their best when facing the world. The new patient is assigned to a hard and unusually high bed, possibly one amongst twenty or thirty others. Screens are temporarily pulled around the bed. He undresses, packs his own clothes so they can be taken away for storage, puts on the hospital garment which has been provided, and climbs into bed. The screens are pulled back and he finds himself an anonymous patient in a hospital ward. The young nurse comes and asks him questions about himself — his age, his occupation, religious affiliation, etc. — which he has already answered to the admissions clerk. The people in the adjacent beds eye him carefully, and they have now heard more details about him than many of his neighbours of years' standing. The young doctor also retraces the questions asked before, plus others about his drinking habits, financial status, ownership or otherwise of his home, family relationships. Those in the adjacent beds now know even more about him because these dialogues are brisk and matter of fact, the information is routine and does not have to be sought in hushed tones. The new patient is left feeling rather naked after these encounters, and this 'personal nakedness' is added to all the anxieties related to the reason for coming into hospital in the first place and those arising from being away from work and home. Without the slightest idea of what they are actually doing and with nothing but the best of intentions towards the patient, the hospital staff are enacting a time-honoured ritual which has the prime effect of reducing the patient as an independent person. Total institutions do not want independent spirits so, consciously or otherwise, they strip away the individuality.

No doctor will easily accept that these practices go on in his own hospital where he has great regard for the kindness and dedication of the staff, but doctors are seldom the best judges of what actually happens as they are seldom about for more than a few hours in the twenty-four. The story *One Flew over the Cuckoo's Nest* by Ken Kesey[6] and the film made of the book, give a painfully close vision of what can happen in hospitals even when staff are moved by the highest motives and the best intentions towards the patients. When we are in positions of authority it is so easy for us to interpret events in a way which serves to strengthen our authority. For example, the high-spirited youth may easily be seen as a trouble-maker when in fact all he has done is to fail to treat those in authority with submissive reverence. The querulous, uncooperative woman is branded a 'difficult patient' because she does not have the mental equipment to discuss her domestic anxieties calmly and rationally with the staff, who are of intimidatingly higher social status.

The stripping process in penal, military and religious institutions is merely the first step, after which the inmate is remodelled in the form desired by the discipline concerned. In hospitals it is only the stripping which is necessary, and it would seem that on the whole the staff do a pretty efficient job. Patients are generally docile and effusively grateful for all that is being done for them. So docile in fact that it is hard for hospital administrators to get any constructive criticisms about the care patients have received so long as they are still in-patients. After discharge, and with skilled interviewers, a totally different picture emerges.

Ann Cartwright[7] a sociologist, interviewed a large sample of patients in their homes after discharge from hospital. She found that:

> Whatever the reasons, patients were more critical about the difficulty of obtaining information than of any other aspect of their hospital care. Whereas only 12 per cent of the patients were not entirely satisfied with their medical treatment, and 23 per cent made some critical comment on the nursing, 61 per cent described some failure of communication.

Of those with communication difficulties:

> 21 per cent said, in answer to a direct question, that they were unable to find out all they wanted to know about their condition, their treatment or their progress while in hospital. A further 5 per cent said they would have liked things explained to them in more detail, another 3 per cent said they were not able to find out about things as soon as they wanted to, and an additional 13 per cent made other comments which indicated that they were not entirely satisfied with the information they received. Finally, a further 19 per cent had had some difficulty in communication, since they had been unable to think of all the things they wanted to ask the doctors while they were there, and only thought of some things afterwards.

But what was it exactly that the patients wanted to know? Mainly, it seemed, details of treatment and prognosis, duration of disabilities, what was going to be done for them and when, the effect on their future sexual and reproductive functions, the significance of symptoms, the purposes of pills. It was sad that patients felt they could not expect explanations, and that some feared a rebuff if they asked. Most of the information that the patients did manage to obtain came from other than the medical staff.

The lack of information patients receive is a direct result of the distance hospital workers place between themselves and their patients, and this distance is a consequence of the conditioning process described as stripping. Only when staff can play down their authoritarian tendencies, manage their organizations as discreetly as possible, and reveal themselves as genuine human beings, will the patients ever feel able to express their personalities and the worries that everyone is prone to who lies ill day after day in a hospital bed. Of course if the patients are given their voice precious time will have to be spent in explanations. Some of the voices may utter criticisms the staff might prefer not to hear. The staff at first may feel less secure. But in the long run a much better atmosphere is established, and, what is more, patients with knowledge in some degree of their condition can participate more in their treatment, and the reduced anxiety can hasten postoperative recovery.[8]

Nurses

The warm-hearted girl enters nursing because she wants to look after people, but she is beset with rules and her initiative is stifled by an inflexible administration. Nursing is caring for sick people, but a profession has been made out of it, life-times are spent in it, so careers must be constructed. Those at the top of the pyramid are often (but not always) there because they did not have the chance to escape. Somewhere along the hierarchy the warm-hearted girl turns into the unimaginative authoritarian. Nurses carry out orders, on their own they can initiate nothing — apart from Florence Nightingale who invented them in their present form. Traditionally they are the handmaidens of the doctors though a Chief Nursing Officer is a powerful person with a salary to match, and with the means to block any enterprise.

Nursing abounds in such paradoxes, probably because the simple direct business of caring cannot easily be profession-alized and incorporated into a technological organization. Nursing makes an unhappy profession. Wastage rates of 40 or 50% are a source of embarrassment, a drain on national resources, and represent a great deal of disappointment, but they are not uncommon. The Manchester Regional Hospital Board were so concerned about their wastage rate — between 38 and 64% in the various hospitals under their control — that they commissioned a special survey. R.W. Revans, who set up the study, found such extraordinary practices in operation with such far-reaching implications for patient care that the results have been published in book form[9] and also in summary in a paper.[10]

He selected 'five acute general hospitals of approximately the same size' for his survey of nurse wastage. At the best hospitals (in this respect) for every 100 nurses completing their training 22 dropped out; at the worst for every 100 completing the course 133 dropped out. The reasons for dropping out might be (*a*) marriage, sickness or rejection by the hospital, or (*b*) a voluntary withdrawal in the absence of any of these factors. Since the drop-out rates for marriage, sickness and rejection by the hospital were similar for the five hospitals, the considerable variations were seen as the results of voluntary withdrawal.

It also emereged that hospitals which could not keep their student nurses had a high turnover of ward sisters, staff nurses, and assistant nurses 'and their record with matrons and domestics was also indifferent'. In these hospitals the nurses also had 'a significantly higher sickness rate', so it would seem that student nurse wastage is only one manifestation of a deeper ailment of the hospital organization. It led Revans and his team to ask whether those hospitals which could not keep their nurses were really able to do their best for their patients. It seemed not. Patients who were in for appendicectomy, hernia repair, cholecystectomy, partial gastrectomy, asthma, bronchitis and pneumonia, stayed on average 50% longer in those hospitals with the high staff turnover.

Revans also found, interestingly, that the average lengths of stay of patients undergoing appendicectomy under four different consultants in hospital X were 8.8, 8.1, 8.5 and 8.1 days, compared with four different consultants at hospital Y where the average lengths of stay were 11.0, 11.2, 11.1 and 11.4 days. This analysis was extended to seven different hospitals and to four different diagnostic groups, and

> . . . in no case did the average length of patient stay associated with any ward, consultant or diagnostic group deviate significantly from the overall pattern set by the particular hospital. The organic tendencies detectable in the hospitals could not therefore be attributed to the idiosyncracies of particular surgeons, particular wards, or particular patients.

Who then could be responsible, because the hospitals

themselves were physically pretty similar? A further investigation was mounted which led to the general conclusion that communications and attitudes up and down the nursing hierarchy were at the root of all the problems so far mentioned. They found that many of the student nurses

> ... could detect little meaning in their daily work patterns ... Many of them ... found it impossible to get explanations of what they were supposed to be doing at all. These difficulties of the girls seemed to be ill understood by those in charge of them, who sought to explain their local difficulties of ward staffing by a decline in the quality of recruits. The survey revealed deep conflicts between the ward sisters and the hospital training staff.

The attitudes of the ward sister to hospital life in general and to the student nurses in particular seemed crucial.

> Individual sisters who had confidence in their superiors displayed sympathetic attitudes towards the student nurses and vice versa; hospitals in which the sisters as a whole had confidence in their superiors as a whole also treated the student nurses as a whole with sympathy.

Revans's findings have been valuable in setting out statistically what many people had suspected for a long time, but it is a survey of large groups, and we want to know more about what the individual nurse may experience. Isabel Menzies, a psychoanalyst, has done this in her study of the nursing organisation of 'a general teaching hospital in London' which she carried out at the request of the administration there.[11] Her starting point was the individual nurse but her conclusions are similar.

> We found it hard to understand how nurses could tolerate so much anxiety, and indeed we found much evidence that they could not ... About one third of the student nurses did not complete their training. Senior staff changed their jobs appreciably more frequently than workers at similar levels in other professions and were unusually prone to seek postgraduate training. Sickness rates were high ...

She lists some of what she calls '*defensive techniques*' which 'the nursing service has developed in the long course of the hospital's history and currently operates'. These defences, she argues, are set up over a long period of time and with little conscious awareness, in order to protect staff from the colossal emotional stresses generated by close prolonged contact with so much human suffering and sadness.

There is a *splitting of the nurse—patient relationship.* Instead of one nurse caring completely for a few patients and doing everything for them, she performs 'tasks' (temperatures, injections, bedpans) for a great many. This practice is defended on the grounds that off-duty arrangements would destroy continuity, and that every nurse should know all the patients on the ward.

Denial of the significance of the individual is epitomized by us all when we speak of 'the liver in bed 10'. But how can any nurse know all 30 patients in a short-stay acute surgical ward? Perhaps the fault lies in the buildings but there has never been great pressure to have the size of the ward unit changed. Then there are the precise regulations governing nurses' uniforms which help to curb individuality among them too. St Thomas's Hospital, London, used to (perhaps still does) require that nurses' skirts hang precisely 14 inches (35 cm) from the floor.

Detachment and denial of feelings. Girls come into nursing around the age of 18 (for eye nursing sometimes as young as 16), and are supposed somehow to nurse bewildered, terrified, pain-racked adults two or three times their age, and perhaps to sustain them through their terminal illnesses. For this awesome task they receive no training, and are simply (and cruelly) told that nurses should be 'above feeling'. A display of feeling regarded as normal in any other setting can bring a reprimand in hospital. Girls come into nursing because of their warm feelings, but they are thrust into a most physically intimate and intense kind of relationship with a severely ill person who needs everything done for him, and then they are abused because they show distress when that person dies. Isabel Menzies comments:

> Seniors showed considerable understanding and sympathy and often remembered surprisingly vividly some of the agonies of their own training. But they lacked confidence in their ability to handle emotional stress in any way other than by repressive techniques, and often said, 'In any case, students won't come and talk to us'.

The weight of *responsibility* that nurses carry for those in their care is so great that in the absence of easy outlet for the emotional consequences of such responsibility it is not surprising that it is frequently side-stepped or simply avoided. Simple tasks, such as bed-making, which can be performed correctly in many different ways, are ritualized, and a virtue is made of uniformity. The endless checking and re-checking of drugs is commendable enough, but not of sheets; and even for drugs a subtle implication is always present that the nurse is not really responsible. After all, doctors do not ask one-another to check the drugs they give in general practice. So strong is the habit of establishing a routine or a ritual for everything (as it is in the army: less so in the air force) that in the end hardly any real responsibility exists in the sense that an individual is able to choose one course of action out of a number of possibilities.

On the other hand there is a general implication that every nurse is directly responsible for the action of every nurse junior to her, so that a third-year student nurse is responsible for what a second-year nurse does, and so on. Since nurses seldom have any clear idea of the range of their duties and responsibilities in the first place this notion of hierarchical responsibility becomes somewhat meaningless, although it could doubtless generate a kind of generalized anxiety from having to bear responsibilities whose scope is never defined.

In such a rigid organization there is an inevitable tendency to resist change. New ideas and techniques generally follow a periodic reappraisal, and, if necessary, rejection, of present practices, but if these cannot be faced squarely little movement is possible. It is a difficult vicious circle to break, and leads to a perpetuation of old habits no matter what outsiders do to bring about change. Nurses often complain that they have no say in what happens to patients although they are the ones who see most of the patients. They may have years of experience but they have to take orders from a doctor qualified last week, or, worse still occasionally, from a newly trained social worker. However, attempts to bring nurses into situations where they will be required to make decisions, such as conducting simple follow-up checks after discharge from hospital, are sometimes disappointing. Anyway, the more independently minded nurses tend to go off into community nursing or health visiting where they have opportunities to function on their own.

Representation on committees and decision-making bodies is expected by many groups nowadays, but in one hospital I know of, when the nurses asked to have access to the committee they were told: 'the Chief Nursing Officer will decide what representation is necessary'. The nurses accepted this ruling unquestioningly.

Deep problems are contained in these examples, and in Britain they have been intensified of late by the reorganization of nursing so that good careers will be possible. The result has been a ten-tier pyramid with a very important Chief Nursing Officer at the top of it, and the tragedy that to make a career of actually nursing the sick is an economic impossibility. Any nurse who wants a reasonable standard of living must fairly early on abandon nursing and take to administration. It is admirable that nurses should partake of the material benefits and have hours of working which will make it possible for them to enjoy them, but nursing the sick is a 24-hour-a-day business which involves a direct relationship between two people sometimes amidst a lot of mess and agony. So far no-one has devised a way of making a high status profession with good career prospects out of this earthy human activity.

Social workers

Social workers are able people who are caught in an even more intractable administrative tangle than the nurses. There are those working in the community who are seen as the traditional providers of child benefits or material comforts for the elderly, and those in hospital who are still seen in the obsolete 'Lady Almoner' image as providing services for the incapable and the needy. To make matters worse an elaborate career structure has been evolved together with the notion that social workers are 'generic', that is they can immediately turn their hand to anything: to acute psychiatric crises, legal questions regarding the care of deprived children, old people's allowances, and so on. This is of course impossible so they have become frustrated at never being able to do anything properly, and to make matters worse they, like the nurses, have an administrative pyramid which only permits the bottom three grades out of eight to have contact with people in need.

Since the social workers are in internal confusion they have not been able to make as great a contribution as they could to medical care, so in hospitals at any rate they are the best educated, most under-used group among the professionals. Furthermore, they have a broad base in the social sciences which makes them objects of suspicion to many doctors who, if they take any notice of them at all, will only allow them to arrange social security benefits and bus fares for their patients. On the other hand they may have a social ease with the doctors which the nurses resent. The nurses may also see social workers as interlopers on hospital wards, which is understandable as the relative role of nurse and social worker with regard to the social care of the patient has never been worked out.

It is quite true that social workers can take over some of the functions of doctors and nurses, and where there is a good personal understanding this is highly advantageous for it allows the doctors more time for exercising their special skills, and the nurses likewise. More than anyone else the social worker can enable the specialist to discharge his obligations to the whole person he is treating. The social worker is better trained than most doctors to enquire into the social background, to sustain bereaved relatives or to make provisions for the family while a parent is in hospital. Doctors who are dimly aware that there is a person behind the hospital patient can lift a great weight off their consciences by learning to work closely with social workers. This need not threaten the doctor's image or status, for it is only in psychiatry that the clinical skills of doctor and social worker overlap.

Social workers are being trained in large numbers and are a major force in community health care at the broadest level. Doctors should do a lot more to integrate them into medical work instead of seeing them as a threat. Although they have a healthy radical disdain for medical elitism, social workers like the rest of the public can be dazzled by the archetypal image of the omniscient physician. Trimming the image down to human proportions so that social workers (and nurses too)

can work as partners with doctors does not always come as
easily as the more liberal-minded doctors might expect.

Professional and technical workers and ancillary staff

Professional and technical workers

There are about thirty categories under this administrative
umbrella of highly skilled and much undervalued workers; for
example biochemists, physicists, psychologists, speech
therapists, occupational therapists, physiotherapists, remedial
gymnasts, orthoptists, chiropodists, dietitians, radiographers,
medical laboratory technicians, dental technicians, cardio-
logical technicians, electroencephalographic recordists, dark
room technicians, hearing aid technicians, medical photo-
graphers, pharmacists, ophthalmic opticians, dispensing
opticians, etc.,[12] and they comprise 6% of the hospital work
force.[1] Most of these have their own professional organizations, training programmes, and a specialized journal
devoted to their activities. They are vigorous within the
hospital; many doctors are almost unaware of them, but the
professional and technical workers are far from unaware of
the doctors, and they form the most discontented group of
all on the hospital scene.[12] There is a widespread feeling that
the complexity of their daily work and the responsibility
they carry is simply not appreciated (or appropriately
rewarded). Because of the way the medical profession is
organized it is the doctors who get all the kudos, and nobody
mentions the technicians without whom a modern hospital
could not function. They feel taken for granted by the
doctors, especially the juniors who give them orders in areas
in which they have considerable expertise of their own, and
they feel it is they who really should be giving the advice and
at times making the recommendations.

This is one area where better communication and understanding of the other's point of view will not necessarily solve
problems. There is too much potential rivalry between
doctors and technicians, and it is made all the more intense
by the fact that many technicians did not get the exams early
on which would have enabled them to train for a medical
qualification. So there is a chronic state of what psychologists call 'sibling rivalry', and that makes great personal

demands on the technicians to accept without resentment the fact that they do have a lower status and lower earning power, and no foreseeable social revolution is likely to change it.

Ancillary staff

These are the porters, domestics, catering staff, works and maintenance engineers, orderlies, laundry workers, etc. who for a long time were a totally silent group, taken for granted rather as faithful retainers of the benevolent institution. More recently in Britain, where the National Health Service is a large pawn in the continuing political struggle, these workers have found their voice and power through trades union organization, so that in the future they will have to be reckoned with and consulted about the general running and development of hospital services. Whether they will become a rogue element or find a satisfying role for themselves in the organization remains to be seen, but since they comprise over one-third of all the people working in hospital they certainly will not be ignored.

Many of the ancillary staff, along with other workers in hospital, have a complicated relationship to the organization and to the doctors in particular, which I suspect contains a fair measure of paternalism. Others simply prefer to work in an environment which is secure and is directed towards doing good. Unfortunately many doctors are currently perceiving these groups as a threat (yet another threat) to their pre-eminence, and are allowing themselves to take defensive stances and to get into conflict yet again. This is quite unnecessary, but they will have to learn to deal on a level with all people working in hospital, to be prepared to justify their own position and to take account of the feelings and opinions of all workers. After all, doctors form only 4% of the hospital work force, and the consultants merely one-third of these.

Summary

Hospitals are extraordinarily complicated organizations which appear to exist primarily for the benefit of the medical staff. Compliant patients are produced by the process known as 'stripping', and although generally satisfied with the quality of medical treatment, most patients are deeply dissatisfied with all matters relating to the communication of information. Nurses, too, are an unhappy group with high wastage rates and styles of organization which are bound to generate anxiety. Social workers, professional and technical workers and ancillary staffs have great importance but still carry relatively low status in the system, so that they are becoming increasingly vocal and militant in hospitals.

5. Patients' Responses to Illness

When the human organism is threatened, either physically or psychologically, various defence mechanisms come into play. Some of these are desirable because they enable the individual to adapt at his own pace to the new circumstances. All of them will have advantages at times. However, they may all become pathological responses if they are allowed to harden into rigid attitudes which no-one can shift.

Individual responses

The responses to be considered here are depression and mourning, denial, displacement, high anxiety and sustained hypervigilance, passivity and regression, invalid role and secondary gain.

Depression and mourning

In illness the body is no longer the intact organism which functions impeccably and never draws attention to itself. It will no longer do all that is asked of it, and the open-endedness of life is gone. The fact that the body — and so life itself — will one day cease to exist becomes an immediate issue. This is not a direct confrontation with death; rather the idea has been introduced that life is finite. Thus the ill person mourns the loss of the intact body and the loss of the illusion of infinite life.

45

Henceforth, the body may not work so well. Activities may have to be curbed, there may be dependence on drugs and visits to hospital to maintain any degree of fitness, there will always be the threat of further deterioration. It is so easy for doctors to say when hurrying to get through a busy clinic: 'Oh yes, you do have some diabetes but you should be able to control it with careful dieting. If not there are excellent tablets you can take . . .' Doctors may talk in the same way to someone requiring replacement therapy, or a colostomy, or who will become dependent on an appliance or a machine, be it a wheelchair, artifical kidney or cardiac pacemaker. But for the patient this means a total reorganization of every aspect of life and the adoption of altogether new routines and goals. Naturally the patient will react profoundly within, but whether the doctor is aware of this suffering depends on whether he tries to listen or else occupies himself with optimistic platitudes about the future.

The initial reaction of the patient is likely to be depression: an almost overwhelming feeling of hopelessness, of the meaninglessness of everything and of the futility of the daily round. There may be resentment against the doctor who gives the bad news, even blaming him for bringing about such a terrible state of affairs. There may be uncomfortable scenes of anguish at the lost intactness of the body, sobbing, clutching, pleading to the doctor to admit that he is mistaken in his diagnosis. It is grief of the same kind as when someone close dies. It is not socially acceptable to grieve for one's body, so it has to be bottled up. But the emotion must be allowed to pour out. It is not the sign of a difficult patient; rather it shows that the patient has perceived the realities of the illness and this is the first step towards a realistic acceptance of life on different terms.

With warm support from the doctor, and every opportunity given for the expression of feelings however intense and abrasive, the 'acute' stage of mourning can be worked through constructively and the patient will become an active participant in this new kind of life.

The responses which follow now are less desirable, and ones which are likely when the initial confrontation with the realities of illness has not been handled well.

Denial

The best behaved patient in the ward can sometimes be the most troubled. The 'good patient' who lies uncomplaining and appreciative in bed, who jokes with the nurses and calls them 'angels' can often be denying ostrich-fashion the realities of his illness. Just as the bereaved often require several weeks before they can accept that a person has actually died, certain people need time before they can accept the full implications of illness. They are letting themselves in gently by the process of denial.

Unfortunately, some people will not on their own come to accept these realities, and they cause problems for themselves and their medical advisers at every stage. They do not come forward in the first place and see the doctor as soon as symptoms have become firmly established. They deny the seriousness of, say, a major operation. They discharge themselves too soon after a myocardial infarct, or they resume active sports while they should be resting to allow diseased tissues to recover their vitality gradually.[1] At this early stage in the patient's journey it is sufficient for the doctor to recognize that he has a denier of reality so as to be on his guard, and also so that he can take every opportunity to introduce the facts about the illness in as much detail as the patient is ready to accept.

It is quite true that some patients get all the way through major surgery, and some get all the way through their final illness and on to death, without ever having faced the truth about what is the matter with them, but these should be a small minority. Too often the argument for allowing patients to deny their illness rests on a failure to understand that the denial conceals a profound distress just below the surface. Also it often makes the doctor's task easier if the patient remains in ignorance.

Displacement

If the illness cannot be accepted by the patient as something which is part of himself, he may react by finding fault with those around him. They may be held responsible in some curious way for the illness itself; more likely they will become the target for all kinds of dissatisfactions related or unrelated to the illness. Complaints about hospital food, the way the nurses make beds or give injections, the habits of other patients, may well be justified, but often such complaints have a petulant quality and an intensity out of proportion to the actual event which should suggest that the real basis for the patient's distress is elsewhere.

Displacement is a common human tendency. It is quite common for someone with a variety of rather intractable personal problems to present with symptoms of anxiety and depression which are entirely blamed on the neighbour's noisy television set. The patient might even say: 'If only I could move to a quieter house then all my problems would be over'. Unfortunately the reality is not that simple for the problem is usually within the individual, and trying to find an explanation outside is not likely to be successful in the long run.

The displacing patient is querulous and argumentative. He objects to hospital routines, questions members of staff about their qualifications for the job they are doing, and tries always to deal with the 'top' person. Unfair comparisons are made with other hospitals and other doctors, and nothing is ever satisfactory where he is. These patients have a way of attracting trouble and seemingly making things go wrong, and so confirming their worst suspicions. Sometimes they may become so dissatisfied that they take their own discharge, which is unfortunate, but it does allow the patient time to come to terms with the reality of illness in his own way, so that he can return to the ward later in a more constructive frame of mind.

The anger should be dealt with for what it really represents, and the superficial criticisms noted but not reacted to emotionally. Staff can remind themselves that they personally are not the target for these verbal assaults but rather it is the professional role which they inhabit. Once the patient comes to feel secure in the care of the staff the difficult habits are likely to subside. If not, it may be necessary to have it out directly, and confront the patient with the realities of his behaviour: 'We are doing our best to help you, but you seem to be continually dissatisfied and finding fault with the staff. Are you really dissatisfied with the care you are receiving? If so, perhaps you could be more specific'. This kind of confrontation will probably be met with a denial of dissatisfaction, and invites the question: 'Why then are you behaving in a way which gives us all the impression that you are?' This should at least clear the air. Even if the patient does not want to talk about his anxieties (though he probably will if given the chance) it will lead to a more open and frank interaction between staff and patient.

High anxiety and sustained hypervigilance

The patient is simply terrified. He sits bolt upright in bed, stiff but starting at every sound in the ward. Sometimes he is visibly trembling. He may be nursing the quiet certainty that he will never leave the hospital alive and will be seeking constant reassurance.

All kinds of circumstances can lead people to become excessively anxious in hospital — operations on emotionally loaded organs such as the heart, the eye and the uterus; operative procedures which threaten the self-image and bodily function such as mastectomy, amputation and colostomy; extraneous psychosocial problems; or associations with the particular hospital or even with the particular ward. Some people, however, are simply of a 'nervous disposition' and tend to react excessively to every crisis, and there are others who allow all the tensions to spill directly out into the open — the very antithesis of the stiff-upper-lip Anglo-Saxon. For these people manifest anxiety, wailing, groaning, even screaming is normal, and, in their culture or family circle, a perfectly acceptable style of response. Not so acceptable in a large ward.

If the basis for the anxiety can be constructively discussed, it is more effective to do this than prescribe large doses of tranquillizers. For the remainder, repeated, and I mean repeated, comforting and reassurance as well as tranquillizing drugs will be inevitable. But it is important for staff to recognize anxiety reactions in their true light, otherwise the staff also become anxious and that compounds the problem.

Passivity and regression

One of the main benefits to come from the winter ailments which afflict so many people is that they provide an opportunity to become passive, to withdraw, to be looked after, and so for a while to regress to the dependent and secure state of early infancy. It is a need which everyone can indulge, and is an important component of all illness.

The organization of most hospitals encourages patients to regress and be dependent, but they must not become too helpless. I feel that patients are allowed to become too passive and acquiescent, and so are not encouraged or allowed to participate as much in the treatment as they are really capable of doing. On the other hand, we must at times recognize the need of certain people to regress, and must accept it and not badger them to make decisions they are not at the time capable of making.

Passivity and regression are mentioned here as examples of adverse reaction to illness. In their more extreme form they become examples of the 'invalid role'.

Invalid role and secondary gain

Nobody likes illness or incapacity, but for many the disadvantages of invalidism are less threatening than full health with all the economic and social responsibilities that come from being a fully able member of society. The temporary regression seen in an acute illness may become a lasting habit in someone with a need for an 'emotional crutch'. For example, 'my rheumatics' become a reason for avoiding all kinds of activities, and a kind of excuse for not being more successful in life in general. This is not to say that such situations are consciously contrived — far from it — and the sufferers would be deeply hurt to think that they were being regarded as malingerers. It is likely that they are people who simply do not, as things currently stand in their lives, have the emotional resources to carry the burdens they used to.

There is another group of people who have coped adequately but who suffer a reverse in their lives after which they never regain their former capacities or self-reliance. They may be people who have coped unusually well, such as a woman who has successfully brought up a large family and launched them into the world. Her husband dies, and she never seems to get over it. She develops a variety of somatic symptoms and makes frequent visits to the doctor, and no amount of medical investigation comes up with any treatable condition. Then there are those who have never coped well but have either been protected by their ageing parents or else by secure employment, until the parents die or they lose their job. I see one such woman who worked satisfactorily for years in a hospital kitchen. Then she was made redundant. She was of low intelligence and could not adapt to her new circumstances, nor could she really cope with independent life in the community. She developed ear symptoms, backache, headaches, phlebitis, and pains in her knees which led her to specialists in different parts of the hospital. Sometimes these specialists would lose patience with her whereupon she would complain to the hospital administration about inadequate treatment. She was referred to the psychiatric clinic, and now ten minutes friendly chat every few weeks about herself, as opposed to her body, has reduced considerably the demands on other departments, which means a worthwhile saving of specialist time, diagnostic resources and useless treatments.

What this woman is getting is in some measure what all people in this category require, and that is someone who will bear their needs for dependency. General practitioners sustain many dependent people but I have been surprised how many hospital specialists do the same. Unfortunately, they can seldom just support people, they have to investigate them and these patients can always offer some new symptom for them to pursue.

The reason for including this group here is to draw attention to the danger of allowing patients inadvertently to slip into the passive dependent role (whether or not they turn out to have some substantial pathology), especially when they are people who have suffered some recent reverse in their lives. Once the invalid role is established it is difficult to shift people out of it as, from the patient's point of view, it represents a pretty good adaptation to their current circumstances. A variant on this theme can be seen in the sufferer from chronic valvular disease of the heart or certain congenital abnormalities when years of incapacity look as though they have been brought to an end by successful surgery. The patient makes a slow functional recovery and may remain passive, although the postoperative studies show a good haemodynamic result. The obligations which come with full health and the loss of dependency are not always so attractive once they have been achieved.

Delay in seeking medical care

Some patients rush to the doctor for the slightest reason but others may use any excuse to avoid attending. Doctors are usually left slightly bewildered by someone who lets obvious disease progress unchecked, especially in a society where medical care is free and there are generous benefits for those away from work. An event — in this case, illness — perhaps cannot be faced in its cold reality, or at any rate it cannot be faced fully and all at once. Defence mechanisms give a person time to adapt, but if a pathological process is continuing during this phase of denial, that is not in the long run to anyone's advantage. For this reason we are interested in those people who delay in coming forward. We want to know how common the problem is, who the people are who delay, and what the underlying psychological mechanisms may be. A group in Cincinatti, working in a hospital where patients would be treated free if they could not afford the fees, endeavoured to answer these questions by taking a random sample of 200 surgical patients. Of these, 166 were not emergencies, and so could have delayed seeking advice: 43% of them did delay. The investigators found that there were no differences between the delayers and non-delayers with regard to age, sex, intelligence or psychiatric history, and all members of this sample were from the 'economically deprived strata'.[2]

They proceeded on the sensible assumption that people will not necessarily be conscious of why they do things, and so instituted a number of in-depth interviews and tests to discover the patient's attitudes to illness and hospitalization. It emerged that 26% of the delayers saw surgical treatment in terms of punishment, and had 'gruesome fantasies' about what would happen to them; 15% had an excessive fear of dying, while 9% delayed because they were depressed and had suicidal wishes. 14% were patients with a self-image that demanded perfect health and the possibility of illness could not be accepted. The researchers thought that some of this group were in fact over-compensating for a deep need for dependency. 13% felt shame about their illness. Most of these patients had illnesses in the genital area, and felt guilt about sexual impulses. 9% delayed because of aspects of their relationship with the referring doctor.

With regard to the diagnoses: 23% of the delayers were found to be suffering from cancer and 32% from conditions involving the genitalia.

Of course these different categories reflect the theoretical standpoint of the investigators (which is psychoanalytic) but the study does emphasize the complex factors involved.

Delay in seeking advice for suspected cancer

A fair proportion of the delaying patients are subsequently found to have cancer. Some workers will state firmly that patients with symptoms which turn out to be those of cancer are more likely to delay in seeking advice than patients with symptoms which turn out to be of general medical disorders.[3-6]

In Boston in 1973, it was found that 34% of cancer patients delayed one month or more before consulting a physician. This compares with a similar study at the same hospital some 30 years previously when 29% delayed, and the figures are not fundamentally different from those collected even 50 years before.[7] This is rather odd bearing in mind the great advances in cancer therapy in recent years, not to mention the huge efforts in the direction of cancer education. At least it is odd if it is assumed that people come forward or fail to come forward with suspected cancer for altogether straightforward reasons. The outlook may be better now than thirty years ago but people's reactions to what is still the most dreaded disease have probably not changed much. Anyway, what sort of people are the cancer delayers?

An approximate profile of the delayer on the basis of various studies[6,8-11] would be: older age group; low social class; little factual knowledge about cancer and feelings that it might be a punishment for past (likely sexual) misdeeds; a tendency to delay consulting the doctor for other medical reasons, together with a related tendency to visit fringe practitioners; pain as a presenting symptom (as opposed to finding a lump or noticing a change in bowel habit); and, of course, having a cancer in a concealed site such as the colon. On the other hand those who come forward early are likely to be: younger; of higher social class; better educated and with a matter-of-fact attitude towards cancer; prone to be active (rather than apathetic) at times of stress; and suffering from cancer in a prominent site such as the breast. Mental disorder does not seem to correlate one way or the other with delay.

The important message to me from these studies of delay is that the way people react to the threat of illness is not rational, and can never be expected to be rational. The attitudes of shame which used to be attached to having tuberculosis persisted for a long time after the disease had been shown to be curable; no doubt something similar applies to cancer. Cancer education and routine screening programmes have not been as successful as on rational grounds they ought to have been. The early appearances are now better known, and are presumably taken in subconsciously by the delayers, but cancer cannot be cured for sure.

It is hard to see what the individual doctor can do about someone who is not there, but when the patient does come forward it is well to remember the deep-seated fears of shame and guilt which may cause added distress on top of the realization that the diagnosis is cancer.

Delay by doctors in diagnosing cancer

So far the patient has been criticised for staying away from the doctor, now it will become apparent that even when the patient does disclose suspicious symptoms the doctor, for various reasons, will not always register them.

A survey of five thousand cancer patients which showed that 38% of patients delayed three months or more[5] also revealed that 18% of doctors delayed one month or more between the time when the patient was first seen and when the diagnosis was made or else referral made to an appropriate agency. Sometimes the reasons will be found in the circumstances of busy clinical practice. Patients will occasionally resent an examination which requires layers of clothes to be removed, and from the doctor's point of view careful physical examinations take up a great deal of valuable time. Some will feel hesitant about performing genital examinations on young patients or on those known personally to them. There is a tendency always to let things slide: if the first examination reveals nothing definite then no further action is taken, or else a remark is made such as: 'We'll keep an eye on it'. Better perhaps to make no examinations at all than foster dangerously misleading expectations.

The Cincinnati group[2] put the problem rather well:

> Sometimes there was mutual hostility between the physician and his patient, with a resulting interference with the normal process of diagnosis and treatment. In other instances strong, positive sympathetic feeling toward the patient irrationally prevented the physician from making a diagnosis with poor prognosis and caused him to act on the basis of wish fulfillment, treating the patient as though he or she had a less serious condition. In two cases in our series the physicians who were close emotionally to their patients treated them for menopausal symptoms when one was bleeding from advanced uterine cervical carcinoma. It was inferred, though not proved, that in each case the otherwise competent physician was too moved by the suspicion of gloomy prognosis to employ his full diagnostic prowess.

It would seem likely that the factors which hold back certain members of the public from coming forward with their suspected cancers also act upon the medical profession. This is a dangerous probability as doctors have many ways of operating the denial processes, and in holding the distressing realities out of reach of themselves they deny the patients the benefit of prompt treatment.

Doctors with cancer

What happens, we may ask, when doctors themselves develop

cancer? They are well placed to select the best treatment from the most energetic and competent clinicians, but what happens in practice?

Of 229 New York doctors and 2000 lay persons who all subsequently turned out to have cancer, just under 40% of each group delayed three months or more before seeking advice.[12] 22% of the medical advisers to the lay group delayed one month or more in reaching the diagnosis or otherwise failed to take appropriate action, which is in line with what we have already seen. But what about the care the medically qualified patients received, these people who ought to be able to chooose the best? Their medical advisers delayed on 19% of occasions – only marginally better than for the lay group. Curiously enough the doctors with superficial cancers, such as of the skin, lip and anterior part of the tongue, delayed about twice as often as doctors with cancers requiring thorough clinical examination or special diagnostic techniques (posterior part of the tongue, rectum, gynaecological cancers, and malignant lymphomas, cancers of lung, oesophagus, stomach, colon, kidney or bladder).

W.C. Alvarez,[13] reflecting in 1931 on the poor prognosis for carcinoma of the stomach, thought that he might get some illumination about how to make an earlier diagnosis by studying the records of doctors who subsequently developed the condition. He picked out 41 consecutive records of doctors who had been operated upon at the Mayo Clinic for cancer of the stomach in the preceding seven years. He was disappointed at what he found. There was, for example, a gastroenterologist of 52 who 'was content to drift along for a year with marked obstruction at the pylorus'. Another, a woman physician, whose mother had died of cancer of the stomach, 'allowed herself to lose 40 pounds [18kg] and go for a year without a diagnosis'.

A series of 60 doctors from the southern United States tells the same melancholy story.[14] Out of twelve with carcinoma of the prostate, eight had metastases when first seen and only two were considered to have had curative operations. Nine with 'upper gastrointestinal tract' cancers all had metastases, as did the seven with lung cancer. Of the nine with 'large bowel' cancers, six had metastases but three curative operations were done. The series included no controls but the author wrote: 'in no instance among those patients with large bowel neoplasm did the physician present himself within the first three months after the onset of some characteristic symptom'.

Whether as doctors we delay more or less than the general population before seeking advice is hard to say from the figures and examples given. But bearing in mind our training and the knowledge we have or at one time did have, our collective behaviour sounds like an active denial of reality — in this case the possibility of death. Of course these studies were mostly carried out some time ago, and diagnostic and therapeutic methods have improved out of all recognition. Doctors have shown that they can heed warnings with benefit, and many will live longer because they have now reduced their consumption of tobacco. However, this was a case which called for decisive action which would bring benefit. Here, we are considering an early sign which may herald death itself. It is this awareness of the possibility of death which triggers the denial mechanism. We should all try to prepare ourselves so that we will not fall victim to fatal denial. Try and generate a fantasy of cancer within. Imagine the sensation of food sticking in the gullet, the feeling of incomplete emptying of the rectum, the shock at seeing bright red blood in the urine. If the fantasy can be held in full consciousness, then the reality can probably be accepted in consciousness also.

Summary

Illness brings forth complex responses from people. These responses, which may be adaptive or maladaptive, are considered under the headings: depression and mourning, denial, displacement, high anxiety and sustained hypervigilance, passivity and regression, invalid role and secondary gain. One of the consequences of these processes is the delay often observed in patients coming forward for treatment. This is explored with special regard to cancer. It is also shown that doctors can be excessively slow at diagnosing cancer, and perhaps slowest of all at diagnosing it in themselves or in fellow doctors.

6. Before the Operation

Ward routines

The six o'clock in the morning cup of tea is not only a perennial joke, it is a continuing reality.[1] No one knows why it needs to be so early. The doctors say that the nursing staff are inflexible in their routines: the nurses say that they have to be ready for the consultant's round, and thus it is a symptom of an uneasiness between the medical and nursing professions which has persisted since the time of Florence Nightingale.

Doctors make stringent demands and they expect a high standard, which is only proper when there are seriously ill people to be cared for. The nurses have to meet these demands with inevitably limited resources. They have to make sure the care of patients continues round the clock, during public holidays, and times of staff sickness. I do not feel that most doctors are aware of, or are particularly interested in, the sheer difficulty of keeping all the nursing routines going in hospital, any more than men in the past were aware of what was involved in running a home. When doctors have plenty of medical problems to exercise them they are disinclined to take on the troubles of the nurses as well.

It is one of those situations to which the contemporary cliché answer is: we want better communication. Unfortunately better communication would not suit all the doctors working in hospitals. If nurses collectively could express all their feelings to doctors, I suspect we doctors would be left feeling that we had the best of the bargain. When we start on the wards, the ward sister holds our hand and stops us making a fool of ourselves. When we become more confident we give her her orders. We breeze into the ward at a moment of crisis, then breeze out again past admiring patients, while leaving the nurses to clear up the mess. We put up with demanding patients for a few minutes before we have to dash off to other things, the nurses put up with the demands for the whole of an eight-hour shift. So often they do the work, and we take the credit (and the income). No, I am not sure whether better communication would do anything but intensify the conflict.

The rigid routines which persist in hospitals I see as a maladaptive response to the nurses' anomalous situation. Because they cannot work in true partnership with the doctors they have set up alternative goals: to run an immaculate ward. Florence Nightingale was determined that the hospitals and nurses in her charge should be above reproach. This was partly in order to get the profession of nursing established at a proper level, and partly on account of her own ferocious personality.

Her approach was highly successful, but it seemed to generate its own momentum so that the high standards of care became an end in themselves, and led to the development of routines which have become exceedingly hard to change except in the smallest degree. I suspect that there will have to be a fundamental revision of the ways in which doctors and nurses view each other's roles, and of the way in which they work together, before the much needed modifications of hospital routine will ever come about.

The ward round

It is hard to write about ward rounds without the descriptions taking on an air of fantasy or farce. The best examples I encountered were in London teaching hospitals. At the Middlesex Hospital, Dr Beaumont's routine arrival would strike the casual onlooker like the visit of a civic dignitary.

The large chauffeur-driven car drew up at the main entrance, the door was opened for him by another official. Walking across the large hall the eminent doctor removed his black hat with his right hand and held it outstretched, to where someone was positioned to receive it, without his having to deflect his gaze or falter in his step. Directly opposite the entrance were the lifts, and the medical part of his retinue was assembled there — senior registrar, registrar, house physicians and students, and also a number of casual visiting students like myself. The qualified doctors entered the lift with the master; the students ran up stairs. At the ward entrance Sister was waiting with *her* staff nurses and student nurses. By the time the medical party arrived there was a crowd of some twenty-five people.

From the clinical point of view, there was of course nothing strictly speaking for the chief to do. The junior medical staff were expected to have seen to that, and they generally ensured that they had done every conceivable test on every patient. There could be no greater slur on the junior's apparent competence than for the chief to ask for the result of a test which he had not thought of doing. The juniors, who were clearly going to succeed in the medical world, often managed to arrange a difficult case or two on which the chief could make a brilliant diagnosis. This might mean that the senior registrar had to be the foil by having overlooked some subtle clinical detail so that his chief could shine, but it was all in a good cause.

Unintentionally, I once became embroiled in this teaching hospital ritual although I did not realize what was going on at the time. The great doctor noticed I was a stranger, pulled me by the sleeve to the front of the group and thrust an X-ray in front of me. It was a film of barium in the duodenum. I recognized that there was a barium-filled pouch on the duodenal wall, which I felt was a reasonable observation to have made. There was then some humourous banter about the ignorance of students from other schools, and one of his own students diagnosed the condition correctly as duodenal diverticulum. He then proceeded to catch out his own students, and his junior medical staff with progresively more arcane questions (always with appreciative laughter from everyone), until he would wink at Sister who was standing there with her entire company of nurses, and say it was time to move on to the next case.

This was a somewhat eccentric round but by no means uniquely so. Where the chief was a clinical virtuoso, like the cardiologist Paul Wood or the neurologist Sir Charles Symonds, ward rounds could be intellectually enthralling, particularly when visiting experts were trying to impress their hosts. Paul Wood, who claimed to recognised 24 heart sounds,[2] was especially good at this. He would lead on a visitor whom he thought was showing too much self-confidence by getting him, say, to listen to the heart of a patient with mitral stenosis. The visitor would find this simple to a degree which made him quite condescending, until he was rendered speechless by his utter inability to say anything to the master about the timing in fractions of a second of the valve sounds or the probable diameter in millimetres of the narrowed valve opening.

The oddest ward rounds are probably farewell rounds. Here the retiring chief treads the wards for the last time, and as many as possible of his past pupils who have reached positions of distinction within the medical profession come to share the experience with him. They proceed from bed to bed in the traditional way but they are quite likely to discuss past patients who inhabited those beds, or else indulge in other reminiscences from the clinics or the rugger field. These occasions can be emotional. St Bartholomew's Hospital bade farewell to two surgeons within a short space of time. One was retiring early to go and grow vines in Portugal, and so was full of zest for his new career: the other who was retiring at the last moment was reported to have been in tears of despair about what he was going to do without his beloved hospital.

There is something grotesque about holding your farewell party in a hospital ward with a compulsory audience of sick people whose attentions are more than adequately occupied with their own travails, and who can have little sympathy for the proceedings. Perhaps there should also be a ward full of suitably grateful former patients to improve the occasion further. A farewell round is a fairly familiar procedure, and it shows just how hospital doctors perceive this function. Ward rounds are staged as though they are intellectual exercises for the improvement of the medical staff. It is as near doctors get to having a regular public platform from which they can demonstrate their professional skills. The ward round is emphatically not an occasion which is designed to meet the needs of the patients, otherwise farewell rounds and humiliating teaching rounds could never be contemplated. Whatever doctors say to the contrary, their attitudes to the patients under their care in hospital are publically proclaimed by the way they act towards those patients.

It is argued that patients can benefit from the bedside dialogues because they hear the relevant facts debated critically by several experts instead of having the single opinion of one sympathetic clinician. True, but the *patient* should be the reference point for the proceedings and if he is not, travesties will occur. For instance, in one hospital a man being set up for liver transplant was the object of intense interest, and I had been seeing him because he was depressed. It was later found that he had a bone sarcoma in his pelvis, and he said to me when I went to see him one day: 'I knew I was done for because the doctors didn't stop at the foot of the bed. They just walked on'. The patient was quite right. Lying ill in bed observing the same scene, with endless hours to learn about every tiny gesture and mannerism of the staff, and with a high level of anxiety which causes meanings to be read into every variation of expression, it is not surprising if a solecism so great as not even stopping at the foot of the bed is interpreted for what it really means. I could only agree with him.

The style of the ward round is determined entirely by the attitudes of the consultant. It is an occasion when the vagaries of his personality will emerge and there is a strong possibility that the negative attitudes revealed will be assimilated by the junior medical staff, and by the nursing staff too. This is detectable, for example, in attitudes expressed towards patients who have been admitted following self-poisoning with drugs, and I have had said to me on such a ward: 'He's taking up a bed, you see. And we've got patients coming in'.

By contrast, I know a number of admirable clinicans in whose retinue a social worker and physiotherapist are more likely to be found than research assistants and visiting academics. They try to avoid working out problems over the patient's supine body by having these discussions before-hand out in the office. Nevertheless, they are never wholly successful from the interpersonal point of view. Ironically, their fascination with clinical medicine keeps breaking through. They make a good contact with the patient, but intense interest is only aroused when a challenging technical medical point crops up. Then they become really alert and get into a kind of huddle with heads forward as they debate the problem with which the patient has obliged them.

When one group of people is incomparably more powerful than another, can there ever be any real dialogue? Even assuming there is good intent from the superior side, can prison warder ever converse deeply with prisoner, teacher with pupil, parent with young child? I do not know, but in the hospital setting I very much doubt it. One group is on its home ground, in its uniform or bearing its subtle symbols of office. Its members have a secure outward place in the hierarchy, however privately anxious they may be. The other group is manifestly anxious about its future. Its members are on strange territory which is difficult to comprehend. They are recumbent and helpless, and more or less depersonalized amongst twenty or thirty sick bodies. They are at such a hopeless disadvantage that all but the most determined will be lulled into a state of passive acquiescence.

How can we redress the balance and strengthen the position of the patient? One suggestion has been that the staff wear the same clothes as the patients, so that the surgeon, instead of putting on a white coat, could put on a pair of hospital pyjamas and sister could cover her dark blue uniform with a cotton nightie. But such a 'levelling down' process is not the important issue. Rather, how can the focus of interest in the ward round be made the patient and not the niceties of disease? This seems to me to be the most pressing question. Some sort of perambulation past patients too ill to get up out of bed seems inevitable, direct observations have to be made upon patients which must then be correlated with information of other kinds so that clinical decisions can be taken, yet we want to keep the individual patient at the centre of this process.[3]

Patients with special problems

There are all kinds of reasons why certain patients should be regarded as being at special risk. Cardiovascular, metabolic and other bodily conditions are mainly outside the scope of this book, and the emphasis here will be on the social and psychological factors, although there can never be a rigid separation. Many of the social and psychological factors have been dealt with in different parts of the book but they will be drawn together here for convenience.

The initial decision to operate must be made in the light of the disordered anatomy or disordered function. This base-line decision can then be modified by various physical and also psychosocial considerations. These factors will, I hope, be introduced not in order to exclude certain patients from the possible benefits of surgery but to highlight where extra support will be needed.

Unfavourable psychosocial background

Problems in this area become immediately obvious to anyone who has the time and interest to sit down with the patient and listen. For the busy doctor they can be assessed conveniently under the following headings:

1. *Bereavement,* by the death of any member of the family or close friend within the past 12 months.
2. *Serious illness or disability* in anyone living with the patient or having to be cared for by the patient.
3. *Problems with the children (if any),* dependent or adult.
4. *Work problems,* actual or threatened, affecting patient or spouse, such as no sick pay, bad working conditions, difficult relations with superiors or subordinates, redundancy or retirement.
5. *Home problems* involving personal relationships in the

home and with neighbours, the building itself, and the immediate environment.

6. *Any other problems.*

This kind of information may modify the initial surgical decision. The quiet patient in bed may be leading a deprived, socially isolated life, with very little money, and an infirm elderly mother who requires constant attention. Coping, for example, with a colostomy or the consequences of a pneumonectomy, could destroy the fragile equilibrium in such a person's life. When psychosocial factors are taken into account the accuracy of prognoses increases substantially.[4]

Previous surgery

A 38-year-old woman was referred to me by a surgeon because she was persistently refusing surgery for a right-sided parotid tumour which was increasing in size. Three years previously she had been pre-medicated and was actually on the trolley waiting to be taken to theatre to have this tumour removed when the operation was unexpectedly cancelled. She had found the experience of pre-medication disorientating and distressing, and she was angry about the cancellation. When seen three years later she was still angry, and although she had kept in regular touch with the surgeon she would not permit him to operate. Not surprisingly to the psychiatrist, there were other personal and family problems. She was clearly aware of these and knowing that she was in a highly anxious state she agreed to come into the psychiatric unit where she received some sedation, and had a chance to talk things over at length. In due course she agreed to the operation (though no pressure was put on her to decide), and it was a complete success since the facial nerve had not yet been affected. There was also a distinct turn for the better in her general attitude to life.

Any previous experience of surgery will be vividly recalled by any patient awaiting operation. It is as well for the doctor to know if this was a tolerable memory or a terrifying one. Any experience of having been a patient in hospital, or even of having had to visit someone in hospital, will be recalled with all its pleasant or sad associations.

Surgery for chronic conditions

Impressive predictions about the kinds of patients who will benefit from surgery for chronic peptic ulcer have been made on the basis of psychosocial data alone[5-7] and the same has been done for open-heart surgery.[8] However, statistical results are not always of obvious help when trying to decide what to do about a particular patient, because we do not want to deprive the patient we know of possible help on the grounds of probabilities relating to patients we do not know. When confronted with the dilemma of finding that the patient falls into an unfavourable prognostic category, the surgeon should follow his instinct but be extra rigorous about his criteria for operating, and also be sure that some kind of social support will be available after the operation.

Those with congenital or other long-standing disabilities will come to surgery as techniques improve. The surgeon's enthusiasm about giving them a new life may not be realized unless a good deal of support is given, and even then it may not be successful, as the transition from invalidism to health involves sacrifices as well as gains.

Emotionally loaded organs and procedures

The heart, the eye, and the uterus are examples of emotionally sensitive organs, but any organ may be sensitive on account of special associations it has for the patient. Similarly, there are sensitive procedures — colostomy, ileostomy, mastectomy, amputation, etc. — and the implications of all these need to be introduced to the patient preoperatively. The most bitter complaints expressed by patients with psychological problems after mutilating surgery arise when they feel they had not been adequately warned of what might happen: when an unexpected colostomy is revealed by the nurse doing the first postoperative dressing; when a permanent suprapubic drain is found when a urinary diversion was anticipated; when a whole breast is found missing although the surgeon had spoken only of removing 'a little lump'.

Psychological problems

Any medical or surgical ward is bound to contain a few patients with psychological problems in some degree, but there are certain specific conditions which will be encountered from time to time.

Intellectual impairment. Many elderly people with failing intellectual powers manage well in familiar surroundings engaged in well practised routines. In the new environment of hospital, with the added burden of illness, and perhaps some degree of toxicity, poor circulation, or any condition leading to diminshed oxygenation of the brain, old people are quite likely to become disorientated because they cannot interpret what is going on around them. Younger people with subnormal intelligence will present the same kind of problem.

Where the deficit is relatively mild, repeated explanation and the presence of familiar persons and objects can reduce their bewilderment so that their management should present no special difficulties, but the surgical operation itself or any change in clinical state could easily precipitate further disorientation. One sure way to generate a crisis is to give elderly patients who are restless and noisy small doses of sedatives, and then isolate them behind screens. This further confuses them and deprives them of what little control they have. Explanation and human contact should precede any sedation, but if drugs are to be given let them be given in doses large enough to be fully effective. The severely subnormal will not ordinarily be treated in general wards.

Manifest mental disorder. There are a number of ways in which a patient may seem to the staff to be mentally disordered. He may relate poorly and seem mainly preoccupied with his own thoughts, possibly giggling to himself from time to time. He may talk out loud as though to someone else, or else express peculiar ideas. He may be deeply depressed, immobile and practically unable to speak without tears rolling down his cheeks, or he may be tediously talkative and jovial. These are gross reactions which are easy to recognize. There are sometimes physical explanations such as the metabolic psychoses associated with vitamin B deficiency or liver failure, or the toxic psychoses due to septicaemia or other toxins such as those in acute pancreatitis, but there are often psychological factors to take into account as well.

For example, a woman of 68 was admitted with acute pancreatitis with a high serum amylase. She was having visual hallucinations, and thought that the nurses were ganging up against her so that she was kicking them whenever they approached her. Her toxic state was quickly brought under control and she was sedated heavily with tranquillizers. When she was lucid again she was able to relate that during the previous year, her husband had been involved in a bad road accident; the day before her son was due to get married there was another road accident in which one person was killed, his future mother-in-law lost an eye, and his fiancée was mildly injured; also, her daughter, with three young children, had had a cerebral embolus which had left her hemiplegic. It is hard to evaluate the relative importance of the physical and psychological factors, and of course it does not alter the management in the acute phase, but I suspect these psychological traumas sensitize a patient, who then becomes more prone than others to develop an adverse psychological reaction.

Psychiatric history. Although the patient appears to be in a good psychological state, it is wise to enquire about any psychological difficulties in the past. 'Have you ever had any trouble with your nerves?' should elicit the necessary inform-ation. As a broad generalization, it is the patient with a long history, with many mental hospital admissions and perhaps a record of antisocial behaviour who is going to be the problem on a general ward rather than someone who had an acute breakdown a few years before and has now evidently recovered, but if in doubt seek specialist advice.

Munchausen syndrome. Richard Asher[9] described what he called the Munchausen syndrome in 1951 and it became an instant success: it was the label that every surgeon and casualty officer had been waiting for to describe a difficult category of patient. Asher was referring to patients who turn up at hospital claiming to be in severe pain, or else with a dramatic history of haemorrhage or the like. They may reveal a multiplicity of scars (usually abdominal) but will be evasive about the origins of these, and their actual clinical state will not accord with the symptomatology. They are often admitted after administration of powerful analgesics but are likely to take their own discharge the next day.

The medical profession, which is always liable to interpret human behaviour in terms of disease, took this basically reasonable description of a peculiar kind of behaviour to be a distinctive disease entity. A fair literature has followed,[10] including an account which claimed to have identified nine varieties,[11] and it has been the subject of a thesis for an M.D. awarded by Cambridge University.[12]

Some of these patients are simply looking for injections of strong analgesics. They may give their intentions away by indicating the drug they feel they require and the route by which it should be given, but many are expert mimics. Simulations of ureteric colic, particularly, can be very convincing.

A much more complex group really do seem to be looking for someone to operate on them — usually on their abdomens. Karl Menninger,[13,14] a psychiatrist, recognized what he called 'polysurgery and polysurgical addiction' back in 1934, but it is hard to make any general statements about these people except that they all have rather disturbed personalities and are submitting themselves to a bodily mutilation which presumably has some special meaning for them. (I have the impression that nurses and would-be nurses are over-represented in this group.) After the abdomen has been opened once there is always a cause of organic pathology for the next time in the form of adhesions, and so with the passage of time and successive laparotomies the clinical problem can become highly complex.

Self-mutilation. Self-mutiliation occurs quite commonly in hospitals for the mentally subnormal, less commonly in hospitals for the adult mentally ill. The form of the mutilation among the subnormal is usually picking, striking, scratching, banging, biting, and with the adult mentally ill also cutting.[15] These people will seldom appear in a general ward, and examples of the practice which surgeons are likely to see will be more diverse. Objects will be swallowed or inserted into any orifice including artifical stomas, and patients will tend to have pretty disturbed personalities. A small number will assault their own genitalia but these people are most likely to be acting in consequence of delusional ideas, probably in relation to guilty feelings concerning their sexuality.

The immediate preoperative period is not the best time to uncover some of the problems just discussed, but the circumstances of surgical life will often make this unavoidable. The surgeon should listen to his own feelings that: 'there's something odd about this patient', and he can ask a social worker or a psychiatric colleague to explore the matter further. From the psychosocial point of view these problems are usually quite straightforward, but the advice and support is likely to be more generally useful if it is sought at an early stage.

Those exhibiting some of the grosser forms of mental disturbance or severe mental subnormality will probably over-extend the resources of the average surgical ward. For them, specialized advice should be sought, but if adequate support can be arranged over the operative period no patient should be deprived of the benefits of surgical interventions on account of psychological disturbance.

Drugs

Such vast quantities of psychoactive drugs are currently prescribed that there is a fair chance that any given patient will be under the influence of some powerful chemical agent affecting the mental state. More and more doctors are now taking a 'drug history' as part of their routine assessment.

Most psychoactive drugs are simply sedative to the central

nervous system, but barbiturates,[17] tricyclic antidepressants,[18] and monoamine oxidase inhibitors[19] can create specific problems as well.

Anticipation of surgery

When a surgical operation is imminent all the patient's attention is likely to be focussed upon it: on the operation itself, on the nature and the extent of the underlying pathology. At this time the simple response of fear will predominate.

Levels of fear

Irving Janis[20] has divided preoperative patients into three groups according to the level of fear they experience in anticipation of the impending operation: high, medium and low. They present in distinctive ways, and more importantly, they correlate with various kinds of adverse postoperative psychological reaction.

High fear patients are restless, tearful, sleepless, hypervigilant towards all activities in the ward, and likely to regard themselves, or to be regarded by others, as hypochondriacal and of a 'nervous disposition'. The prospect of surgery may arouse fantasies of mutilation or annihilation, that the surgeon might make a fatal slip at operation, that too much anaesthetic might be given, or that the heart might stop. They will seek, and will benefit from, repeated reassurance on these and other points, and will also benefit from the use of tranquillizers.[21]

After the operation the same pattern is likely to continue, and patients may doubt that they are, in fact, recovering. However, they will cooperate with the staff, and will express sometimes extravagant gratitude and admiration, but they will demand a good deal of attention because of their tendency to regress to a state of child-like dependence. In short, they are highly anxious people who need a great deal of propping up before and after operation, but with that support there should be no further psychological problems.

Moderate fear is realistic fear. This group have compre-
hended and more or less adapted to the prospect and implications of the operation ahead of them. Certainly they
display apprehension but that is a proper response. They have
anxieties but not to a degree that they cannot take in and
benefit from explanations given by the staff. After the
operation they continue in the same way, and present no
special problems.

Low fear patients were the surprise group in Janis's study.
These are the relaxed and uncomplaining 'good patients'.
They admit to no worries about their condition or about the
operation which is ahead of them, and express great confidence in the skill and competence of all the staff. They are
of course the same group as tended to deny the realities of
their illness when it first became manifest.

After operation the realities will be painfully evident, and
the defence mechanism of denial may not be strong enough
to hold these realities at bay. Defence mechanisms are there
for a psychological purpose, and if they are in danger of
being broken down their possessor is likely to become
severely distressed. This distress may reveal itself in the
postoperative period by moodiness, lack of cooperation in
routine procedures, and even outbursts of belligerent protest.
From being placid and uncomplaining they can become
exceedingly frustrating to the ward staff as nothing that is
done for them is right.

Some of this trouble can be avoided if the patients with a
tendency to deny realities can be recognized before
operation. A patient who seems indifferent to the prospect of a major operation should be given a change to describe what he knows about his condition, and to talk
about his true feelings concerning the operation to come. If
the answers are bland and uninformed, then some effort
should be made gently to confront him with the realities. He
may be able, however reluctantly, to face some of them, and
so graduate to the moderate-fear group. Alternatively, he
may crumple completely and become highly anxious, or depressed, and so need some more time until he will be ready to
face surgery. Yet again, his defences may simply stiffen up,
and no reasonable statement about the realities will have any

effect. A blunt disclosure by the doctor about the presence of potentially fatal disease may be answered simply by the patient discrediting the doctor's competence. Many people find certain truths about themselves too threatening to contemplate under any circumstances.

A number of other investigations have been made into the relationship between preoperative mental state and post-operative progress,[22-24] but one[25] reached an opposite conclusion to Janis in that those of the sample who denied the realities did better than those who tried to face them. These authors claimed that such patients spent less time in hospital postoperatively, required fewer analgesics and had fewer negative psychological reactions or minor physical complications. Their sample on the whole suffered from less serious surgical conditions than Janis's and when their relatively more ill subjects were selected out these authors were less sure of the advantages of denial. So there is no simple answer to the question of how much any given patient ought to know before operation, and I doubt if we shall get one from statistical inquiries.

There is abundant evidence that people want to know what is the matter with them, and some of the work on this subject will be reviewed in Chapter 10 in connection with those who are incurably ill. It is also implicit in any relationship where trust is important that fundamental information is not withheld. If patients are in ignorance of what is going on they can only play the part of passive victims, and are deprived of the chance to participate in the process of treatment.

There was a simple but telling study conducted by anaesthetists and surgeons at the Massachusetts General Hospital[26] in which two comparable groups of patients underwent elective intra-abdominal operations. The study group were given information about what to expect after a surgical operation and what they could do to help themselves. They were told that they would feel pain, how severe it might be and how long it would probably last. It was explained that it was quite normal to feel pain after an operation, and that much of it was due to contractions of the muscles under the incision, and that they could ease it by learning to relax those muscles. They were also shown how to hoist themselves up on the trapeze overhanging the bed, and how to turn on to one side using their arms and legs while relaxing their abdominal muscles. Finally, they were told that at first they would find it difficult to relax completely, and if they could not achieve a reasonable level of comfort they should request an analgesic. The study group were given this information with enthusiasm and confidence: the control group were told nothing about what pain they could expect after operation.

The surgeons and other doctors, the nurses and the patients themselves were unaware that a study was being conducted, and so the administration of postoperative analgesics and other routines up to and including discharge proceeded in the ordinary way. The results are as simple as the experimental design: the study patients required half as much analgesic medication as the control group, and on average they were discharged home by the surgeons almost three whole days earlier than the controls.

Summary

Rigid ward routines and doctor-orientated ward rounds are briefly considered. Then, various psychosocial problems which will be met with frequently amongst preoperative patients: unfavourable psychosocial backgrounds, those who have undergone surgery before, and those with chronic conditions. The issue of emotionally loaded organs and procedures is summarized, plus an account of certain specific psychological problems, intellectual impairment, manifest mental disorder, those with a psychiatric history, the Munchausen syndrome and the self-mutilators, alcholic patients and those taking psychoactive drugs. Lastly the mental state of the patient awaiting operation is described in relation to levels of fear experienced — high, moderate and low.

7. Postoperative Care and Intensive Care

As the sutures go in at the end of the operation and the covering sheets are removed, the supine body begins to stir, tubes are withdrawn, and the person is reappearing once more.

In some ways it is like being born all over again. To begin with there are fumbling movements and a dimly perceived world because of the clouding of awareness by opiates. A total helplessness which makes doctors shy, and in which nurses come into their own. An earthy existence for several days with intimate physical contact with the nurses, and physiotherapists too, where all bodily processes are open and shared. The first steps seem such a triumph, and more pride when steps can be taken without the supporting arm. Advice is sought about everything: when to get dressed, when to bath, if it is possible to walk beyond the ward, and ultimately when to go home.

The surgeon's job is to perform the operation. Thereafter, he and the other doctors on the team merely monitor the patient's progress because their time is taken up selecting and operating upon the next lot of patients. They thereby miss much of the patient's experience of getting well. An operation is a landmark in anybody's life, and the period of recovery can be a fertile time in which the patient — temporarily absolved from the responsibilities and demands of life yet now free from the fears that must precede any operation — can take stock and perhaps reorientate his lifestyle in various ways. Less fortunate people will find no relief from their outside problems and some will find their world contracting down to the boundaries of their hospital bed as they wrestle with the realization of having an illness which cannot be cured. However, this chapter will not pursue the process of uncomplicated recovery or the course of those with incurable conditions (Chapter 10 will) but rather some of the hazards which may befall the large middle group.

Early postoperative period

The patient wants to know if the operation was a success, and anyone may be asked: the hospital porter who pushes the trolley back from theatre, the junior nurse who accompanies the patient on his journey, the orderly waiting in the ward. They will quite properly answer in platitudes but somebody at some stage has got to explain in intelligible terms whatever it has been decided is going to be explained. In other words, some policy is needed: a decision has to be taken about what is to be said, when, and by whom. When the issues are presented in these terms it seems self-evident that the task should be taken on by the surgeon who performed the operation, but it seldom is, and that is quite an interesting question in itself. Why should the surgeon who decides to do the operation in the first place, who goes on to perform it, and who subsequently must have an interest in the outcome, so often feel that it is no concern of his to go and talk things over with the patient?

Of course the surgeon is busy but it says something about his perception of his job that he does not rate talking to patients after operation high on his list of priorities, because all senior hospital doctors have sufficient control over their work schedules to include anything they feel is important. Perhaps the surgeon feels that postoperative care — beyond the management of complications — is the concern of his juniors, and that he has graduated from such tasks. This is understandable because talking to ill people who may be in pain is time-consuming and involves becoming tranquil and receptive, in contrast to the bustling style which gets him through the rest of the day.

Talking to a person whom one has operated on is not as simple as non-surgeons may think. There is an explicit responsibility because one has done some pretty drastic things. Decisions have had to be taken, sometimes quickly during the operation itself, which will have a fundamental effect on the quality of the patient's future life. Some surgeons feel they cannot maintain their ability to make calm, detached and at times ruthless decisions if their intellectual processes are to be complicated by personal considerations. This is a completely understandable attitude but it is not inherent in the nature of surgical practice; rather it suggests that the surgeon has difficulty in handling the feeling component of his work.

What can be expected of all surgeons is that the question of what to say to the patient is openly discussed, and that a definite policy is established for each patient. If not, patients will be needlessly confused and distressed, as was one general practitioner after he had had a lumbar disc removed:[1]

> The expected instant relief of sciatica did not take place. I received four totally different explanations for this worrying and persistent pain — all on request — one suggesting ischaemia of the nerve, one hyperaemia of the nerve, another operative trauma, and yet another adhesions: a fifth was also offered, namely that I did not in fact still have a pain. The surgeon simply said — from the end of the bed a few hours after the operation — that I would be 'none the worse for that', a remark open to many interpretations.

Postoperative complications

Having done everything possible in advance of the event, which is where the effort is most efficiently directed, the postoperative support to the patient can be directed along two lines: first, to keep up morale and encourage the effort to get well, and secondly to try to reduce anxiety and muscular tension. It is assumed, of course, that adequate analgesics and all the usual postoperative measures will be available.

The patient's *morale* depends much on the morale of the nursing staff (as was shown by Revan's comparative survey[2] of hospitals which was discussed in Chapter 4 in connection

with nurses), but what the doctor can give at this stage is
time: time to listen carefully to discover what is uppermost
in the patient's mind, and above all to listen for the unasked
question. Time also to explain and to explain again. Then to
give positive advice about how to cope with each stage of
recovery in hospital and outside. The best way to learn about
recovery from surgical operations is to have one oneself.
Short of that, talk to former patients about their experiences
at different stages, or else ask general practitioners.

The essence of postoperative care from the psychological
point of view is contained in the simple findings of Lawrence
Egbert and his colleagues[3] with which the last chapter ended.
They said in effect that ill-informed patients experience more
pain and recover less rapidly than do well-informed ones.

Anxious postoperative patients are likely to hold their
muscles in a higher than normal state of tension,[4] and the
same goes for persons developing inguinal hernia.[5] These
patients might then be liable to hold themselves stiffly, and
so be unable or disinclined to move much in or out of bed;
in other words the opposite to what is hoped for in the
postoperative patient where mobility is assumed to reduce
the incidence of chest infections and venous thrombosis.
High muscle tension may also place a greater traction on the
healing wound, and so favour disruption. Anxiety and fear
are likely to evoke adrenergic responses in the autonomic
system which could favour the development of retention of
urine or adynamic ileus and perhaps also lead to alteration
of the blood supply to the skin which could further impair
wound healing and resistance to infection. In practice, of
course, these autonomic responses are complex and their
precise modes of functioning are not clearly understood,
therefore comments about these processes must be tentative.

There is sometimes a confusion between anxiety (call it
mental tension) and *muscle tension*. They are not the same,
and reduction of anxiety does not necessarily lead to
muscular relaxation, nor indeed will relaxation exercises
necessarily do this either.[4] The only way I know of to
produce muscular relaxation is by biofeedback techniques,[6]
and no doubt biofeedback devices will gradually make their
way into hospital wards.

Postoperative mental disturbance

A surgical operation, like any other major event in life, may be associated with some kind of psychological difficulty. In addition, the causative illness itself and the disturbance of the operation can introduce chemical, metabolic, toxic, and other factors which can further increase the likelihood of trouble.

Any kind of psychological reaction is possible. Those who become *highly anxious* are generally those who were highly anxious preoperatively, or else who have had distressing experiences in connection with the hospitalization such as frustrating delays, patients dying nearby or repeated painful procedures. Also repeated surgery for the same or for different conditions can lead to an increasing brittleness and lack of tolerance to the inevitable uncomfortable post-operative routines. *Depressive* reactions are also quite common, either as a different kind of response to the types of experience just described or, more likely, as a consequence of serious or incurable disease.

The *acute postoperative psychosis* is the reaction which is going to exercise the hospital staff most. For the first few days after a major operation the patient is likely to be fairly prostrated physically in addition to being sedated by drugs, so nothing much may occur. Three or more days after operation, certain odd behaviour may be noticed: plucking at the bedclothes, making suspicious glances and odd incomprehensible remarks, and wandering attention as though the person is preoccupied with his own thoughts. Food is rejected for no apparent reason, the patient refuses to talk to members of staff, and may deny ever previously having seen the nurse who has been in daily attendance, and fail to recognize close relatives. Sometimes staff may be mis-recognized as members of the family or the like. This odd behaviour may become explicable if the patient gives vent to paranoid ideas, such as the belief that the ward staff are trying to poison him, or that there is some complicated plot afoot to destroy him. There may also be a preoccupation with apparently meaningless but harmless ideas, and also on occasions auditory and visual hallucinations. (These last of course are a common feature in delirium tremens and to a lesser extent in some drug withdrawal states which can manifest themselves postoperatively after emergency surgery, especially for trauma.)

These acute psychotic states may appear gradually, or they may burst forth suddenly when everything seems to be going well. Occasionally the problem may be predominantly psychological since the physical disturbance has been slight; more often a number of different factors have to be taken into consideration.

A 52-year-old woman became severely agitated, disorientated and visually hallucinated some thirteen days after a small bowel resection for volvulus. Most of the time her speech was incoherent but she seemed to be preoccupied with the idea that: 'I'll be punished if I decide'. So on no account should she make any decision. She was seriously ill physically at the time so there was little scope for decision-making but that did not alter the great distress she was experiencing. Unfortunately she was too far into her psychotic state for anyone to reach her and she was delirious from toxicity from bacterial infection. She was also dehydrated and suffering from severe electrolyte imbalance, and these conditions probably worsened in the days before the manifest psychological disturbance when she had quite likely been refusing food and being generally negative. The picture was also complicated by previous illness and surgery. Ulcerative colitis had been diagnosed two years previously, she had developed a rectovaginal fistula after repair of rectocele, had a deep-vein thrombosis, and seven months before the present operation had had a subtotal colectomy for Crohn's disease which had left her with an ileostomy. In addition she was on steroids, and had some collapsed vertebrae thought to be due to this medication.

The nursing and management problem was therefore considerable, and because of her restlessness and resistance to ordinary doses of sedative drugs, her abdominal wall became excoriated from the small bowel contents. Although her toxic state, dehydration and an electrolyte imbalance were quickly corrected it was some five days before she became lucid again, but once she began to improve physically and psychologically she made an uninterrupted recovery, and continued in good health. She was managed on the psychiatric ward but, of course, in close collaboration with the surgeons. With hindsight in this and other similar cases it is difficult to point to one cause since there are so many contributory factors: the psychological distress at repeated surgery, bacterial toxicity, the dehydration and electrolyte imbalance, and possibly the steroid medication as well. All that can be done is to correct everything physical that can be corrected and to see that the patient is nursed by nurses who can relate supportively to someone who is in common parlance 'raving mad'. The success of this case certainly depended on the presence of nurses who were skilled in both surgical and psychiatric nursing.

There is a big literature on postoperative psychoses[7-11] which reflects changing attitudes to these conditions. It has now been superseded by an even bigger literature on the psychological sequels to open-heart surgery.[12-16] Operations on the heart with cardiopulmonary bypass take longer to perform than most operations in general surgery, and they are physically and psychologically more upsetting to the patient. They can also be associated with more severe biochemical disturbances, and cerebral lesions from microemboli, and so there is a complex collection of physical and psychological difficulties. This is further complicated by experiences which may be endured in the postoperative environment.

Special hospital environments

Mechanical, electronic and other technical advances in life-support systems and treatment have led to the creation of special departments in which these measures can be deployed. Great advances have become possible because of these environments, and many people survive who would otherwise have succumbed, but in the process unexpected psychological pressures have been generated which can enact a toll on patients and staff alike.[14]

Broadly speaking these units fall into two categories: those placing the patient in isolation, and those where intensive care is practised.

Isolation units

People may be isolated to prevent infection getting out, as in the case of the traditional isolation ward, or else isolated to prevent infection getting in. In the second category will be those whose immune responses have been suppressed in connection with organ transplantation or cancer chemotherapy, and the isolation for such people can be absolute. They can be touched only through plastic gloves at the end of plastic arms built into walls or by individuals dressed in 'space suits' wearing gloves.[17] Thus there is none of the direct human contact or warmth (perhaps for several weeks on end) which is such an important source of comfort and support, especially to someone who is ill.[18]

Personal isolation. In ordinary hospital wards people can be isolated in single rooms, or even in the open ward when the curtains are pulled round the bed and side rails erected. After cataract extraction and other eye operations which require a period of postoperative blindfolding an even more severe isolation is imposed.[8,19,20]

Isolation can lead to personal distress, and in a number of cases to the kind of acute postoperative psychotic reactions already described. The lack of sensory stimulation because of diminshed input or because of the monotony of the input, and the lack of human contact, is in itself a potent factor in producing disorientation and psychotic-type behaviour, as a great deal of experimental work has shown.[21-24] When sick, elderly (like most cataract patients), and anxious people find themselves in such conditions they are even more likely to succumb than the healthy subjects of experiments.

Intensive care units

These include postoperative recovery rooms for open-heart

and other major surgery, coronary care units, respiratory units, and the general intensive care units which exist in most large acute hospitals. All kinds of people can turn up in them. Waking up in an ICU may be the very first indication that something serious has happened, such as a major accident; alternatively it might be the first tangible step towards health after years of incapacity from heart disease. The patient may be the object of intense therapeutic attention or may simply be there for close observation.

The psychological pressures generated by ICUs have been widely studied[25-27] and as a result they are less disturbing places than they used to be but these pressures can never altogether be removed. I feel I can best illustrate the problem by caricature.

The patient looks around at the white room. Before his operation he had been in a ward with colours and all kinds of faces but now everything looks the same. The lights are bright and there are brilliant surfaces. The moving figures are all in white, and they make no sounds. On the beds are various human shapes, young and old: with emaciated limbs, immense scars, shaven heads, exposed genitals, and tubes and wires connected to them. Some of them move a little, and gasp and groan, and the white figures attend to the yellow, clear or red fluids that run in and out of them. Also there are the lights which flash to reveal the workings of hearts and lungs. Some of the machines make noises too: the respirators click and 'whoosh', suction pumps throb and gurgle, oxygen hisses, and motors hum.

Day follows day. There are windows but they are white panels with nothing beyond. No-one there can eat so there can be no meals to punctuate the day/night. There is no set time for anything because there can be no routine where every moment is crisis or potential crisis. Vistitors come and go. They, too, wear white but they can be distinguished from those who work there because they sniff and sob, and are sometimes led away weeping.

One of the calm gowned figures suddenly dashes to the telephone and sounds a noisy alarm. Within seconds a stampede has started, and all kinds of people without masks burst into the room and make for one of the recumbent figures. They look at the monitor screen and at the eyes, and then lunge on top of the figure who then disappears from view for all the people around the bed. Something highly professional is going on, staff move rapidly and economically, and after a while they all leave, and the figure is once more alone on the bed. The staff are a little more animated for a while, then the calm returns. This ritual happens quite often, and people seem to come and go from the beds. It is hard to be sure of this as the usual features for recognition such as the face are seldom clearly visible, so it is difficult to tell who is who.

People do not have time to linger, and it is clearly tedious trying to understand a question or a remark from someone who has a tube in his windpipe. It is disturbing that every movement causes the heart beat to stagger drunkenly on the monitor screen, and there is a feeling occasionally of floating out of one's body, and then at times terrible feelings of people under the bed or that the tubes are running deadly poison into the body. Someone always comes immediately the bell is pressed but they seem then to go away equally quickly. They supervise everything: the exact number of pillows and the precise angle at which the body should be positioned, the number of spoonfuls of food and the volume of liquid going in and out. Nothing is left to chance or to personal choice. One day the tubes are taken out, and a porter wheels the bed out of the special room back to the surgical ward where everyone is recognizable, where decisions have to be made again and no one bothers about all the details which had seemed so important the day before.

Any intensive care unit can (and the earlier units certainly did) put psychological pressures on the patients which they cannot handle, and the conditions which lead to them being admitted to such units in the first place are all likely to impair their coping ability further. A great deal has been done to ease the lot of patients in ICUs and the former high rates of psychotic reaction[28] should not now occur, but however good the design no one can ever have a completely smooth emotional passage through an intensive care unit because a life-threatening condition is a requirement for entry in the first place. It may be reassuring to be in an ICU but not reassuring to need to be in one.

Patients in intensive care. Lack of response does not mean that a person cannot hear or understand: helplessness is not to be equated with stupidity.

Most experienced doctors have been embarrassed by a patient relating back remarks which had been made over that patient's supposedly unconscious body. Hearing is probably the last faculty to be lost and the first to return, and it is a good working principle to assume that every patient, however apparently badly brain-damaged, can hear and understand what is being said in his presence.

Relating to the unresponsive is a knack which ICU staff have to pick up. They also learn to 'speak in commentary'[29] to patients with tracheostomies. This is a kind of conversation in which the nurse speaks for both persons, and the patient is enabled to join in merely by making the appropriate nods and grunts, but a certain experience and imagination is necessary to anticipate the questions the patient would ask if he could. The machines need to be explained as soon as possible, and they may even be personalized as 'your watchman' or 'mechanical guardian angel'. Similarly terms like 'feeding line' and 'TV set watching your heart beat' along with a great deal of positive reassurance can bring comfort and reduce the anxiety from uncertainty in the strange environment.

On the whole patients tend to look back on their experiences in the ICU with satisfaction. Part of this may be due to the processes of denial of realities where, for example, in a survey of 332 former ICU patients 27% said that they had never been in such a unit at all and even amongst those who had a basic awareness of having been in one, the details, such as whether or not they had been ventilated, were often inaccurately recollected.[30] Some observers have even suggested that denial may improve the survival rate in a coronary care unit.[31]

Transfer away from intensive care can present problems, especially for patients in a coronary care unit since they are liable to feel the separation from the monitors more acutely than the general ICU patients.[25] Appreciable numbers may become depressed or anxious after such transfers (and there may be increased catecholamine excretion) but these undesirable occurrences can largely be avoided by proper preparation for the inevitable — and possibly abrupt — transfer out, and by the provision of a continuity of medical and nursing care.[32,33] The monitors and life-support systems have to be presented to the patients as important but *temporary* aids.

Relatives of patients in intensive care. Grief, anger, guilt and frustration can be felt simultaneously by helpless relatives as they witness the patient being processed by the hospital. The staff will allow them free access, their presence may help the patient keep his psychological bearings, but they can easily become another burden for the staff. They can also communicate their anxieties to the patient, and both patient and relatives can become exhausted by prolonged bedside encounters when no real communication is possible.

Relatives need some explanation before entering an intensive care unit, not only concerning their relative but perhaps also about neighbouring patients whom they cannot avoid noticing. Also, if there is a great pressure of pent-up emotion it would be desirable to allow some of it to be ventilated away from the unit before visitors come face to face with the patient, and then at intervals during their stay there. Hostility and suspicion may be expressed by relatives towards members of the unit staff which may be manifestations of their feelings of distress and helplessness, and they may even suggest that other patients are receiving more than their due share of attention.

Nursing staff in intensive care units. Intensive care nurses have more responsibilities than their colleagues on the general wards, they handle expensive life-saving equipment, but such equipment if mis-used is always in danger of being life-threatening. They have a higher standing with regard to the doctors, and a closeness can develop between doctor and nurse from working most of the time in an atmosphere of crisis. This can lead to a certain separateness of intensive care staff since others will not always appreciate their particular tensions and problems, and so off-duty they may prefer to unwind with other intensive care workers. Staff on extra-specialized units, such as those for renal dialysis[34] or burns,[35] can also have problems in connection with the particular pathologies involved.

The emotional rapport with patients is in some ways weaker than on ordinary hospital wards because the patients are often prostrated or else unable to communicate freely. On the other hand there is a great physical intimacy and a total dependence upon the staff for survival but it is a relationship which is always liable to sudden rupture. The empathic relationship has to be more conscious and more controlled than usual if the wounds of the frequent deaths are not to become overwhelming. A great actor playing *Hamlet* or *King Lear* five times a week could not keep going for long if he had to live out all the emotions encompassed in the play. His technique enables him to give a feeling performance yet keep those feelings separate from his person.

Long hours of resuscitation work, especially at night, amid all the blood and débris of used equipment can take on a dream-like quality in which the harsh fact of people dying becomes blunted, and the distinctions between living and dying seem almost to disappear; at any rate they lose their emotional tone. After a failed and messy postoperative cardiac resuscitation at the Brompton Hospital in London, I sometimes used to go out for a walk into the streets. The contrast between busy South Kensington and the surroundings of the previous hours could engender a surrealistic feeling which was quite agreeable in its way now and again, but I think I would have found the tension of the two intense realities of exuberant life and messy death rather difficult to hold on a regular basis.

Staff will adapt to any amount of horror but the kind of defensive detachment which is necessary when doing military surgery is not desirable in an ordinary civilian hospital. The staff have of course chosen to work in intensive care, and many have individual modes of adaptation which work well for them but what really matters is that the team works well. Flexible duty rotas and a staff room away from the sight and sound of the patients are welcomed, but more and more staff are now having a chance to meet in groups.[36] Here nurses, doctors and other staff can meet together with a leader who is familiar with the work but separate from the actual unit, and together work through the problems and tensions inherent in intensive care. More specifically, the staff learn that the inevitable hostilities, uncertainties, self-doubts, and personal fears can not only be expressed in front of those whom they concern without causing disruption, but they can actually bring working colleagues closer together. Personal distress in relation to particular cases has to be held back at the time but it can be ventilated freely and worked through in the company of the group. Innovative ideas and administrative issues similarly can be discussed. Altogether such meetings should prevent people having to hold the emotional tensions of intensive care work exclusively within themselves.

Summary

Anxious and frightened postoperative patients hold their muscles tense and may produce adrenergic responses, all of which may be associated with the incidence of postoperative complications. Acute postoperative psychosis, which is most common after open heart surgery, is due to a combination of physical and psychological factors. Special therapeutic environments now exist in most large hospitals which can impose psychological pressures on patients either through the isolation imposed or as a result of intensive, 24-hour-a-day care. Staff and relatives also can suffer in these unusual conditions.

8. Pain

Pain as a conscious experience

Any psychosocial approach to pain assumes that pain is not simply the body's response to a certain kind of stimulus, but rather that it is a conscious experience. An unconscious person withdraws his foot following a pin prick, but that is a response to a noxious stimulus, not to pain. Before there can be a sensation which can be called pain there must be consciousness; the person's mental state, previous experiences and cultural attitudes will all come together in determining what is or is not to be regarded as pain; and further how this experience is to be conceptualized, and what kind of response there will be.

Because of the cardinal importance of pain as a symptom in clinical medicine, and because elaborate (although disputed) physiological processes have been described, doctors tend to assume that pain must be the consequence of a physical stimulus. They even go further and regard the stimulus and the experience of pain as the same thing. Many doctors may recognize the association between psychosocial disturbances and exacerbations of a patient's pain, and it may be acknowledged that the pain does not conform to any familiar pattern, but there is still a great reluctance to look for other than physical models of explanation. One good reason for this reluctance is that some obscure treatable physical condition may be at the bottom of it, but a more telling reason is that the great majority of doctors find it

conceptualize pain except in terms of bodily
 ...ere is simply no other way to think about pain
 ...work of orthodox medicine except as something
 ... which must be eliminated. As Ivan Illich has put
 ...tional] culture makes pain tolerable by integrating
it   a meaningful system, cosmopolitan civilization
detaches pain from any subjective or intersubjective context
in order to annihilate it'.[1,2] While one may not accept all
Illich's views on the benefits of pain, he is certainly right in
suggesting that the medical profession has gone too far in the
other direction through its over-simplified view of the nature
of the pain experience. It can lead to absurd situations in
which doctors will tell patients, when they can find no
explanation for a pain in terms of disturbed anatomy or
physiology, that they do not really have pain, or else that
they must be imagining it. This mixture of arrogance and
ignorance can be distressing to patients, and it is as unjus-
tifiable as a doctor telling a patient that he could not possibly
be in love or be feeling sad. Pain is a subjective experience,
and so if people complain of pain it must be assumed that
they are experiencing something they themselves regard as
pain.

Cultural and individual differences in response to pain

Whatever people may actually experience, there are certainly
differences in the way people from various cultures respond
to pain. This will be determined partly by the meaning they
ascribe to their experience, and partly by the social attitudes
to the expression of emotion. However, some of the cultural
differences can be so great as to give food for thought about
the nature of pain itself. Ronald Melzack[3] cites such an
example from a culture in which

> A woman who is going to give birth continues to work in the fields
> until the child is just about to be born. Her husband then gets into
> bed and groans as though he were in great pain while she bears the
> child. In more extreme cases, the husband stays in bed with the
> baby to recover from the terrible ordeal, and the mother almost
> immediately returns to attend to the crops.

Even among the population of a single country, although it contains people of different ethnic backgrounds, great differences in response have been observed in the extensive literature on the subject. Age, sex, race, the state of the autonomic nervous system, carbon dioxide tension in the blood, the presence of nausea, fatigue, anxiety or fear, deliberate distraction from the pain or training in methods of enduring it, emotional excitement such as in battle or in a football match and, of course, drugs have all been shown to alter the response to pain.[4-6] In addition, just about every psychiatric syndrome has been claimed to have some special relationship with the experience of pain.[7,8] It is difficult therefore to reach any general conclusions about the experience of pain, and more profitable really to concentrate upon the individual, to discover what pain means for the particular patient and the part it plays in his life as a whole.

Psychogenic pain

An appreciable proportion of patients with psychogenic pain are depressed.[9,10] An appreciable proportion of depressed patients complain of pain for which no physical basis is found.[11] In surveys of general practice and hospital out-patients substantial numbers of those presenting with pain turn out to have no physical basis for it.[11,12] It would be helpful therefore to discover some way of distinguishing those whose pain is psychogenic from those who have organic pathology.

This challenge was taken up directly by a psychiatrist and a gastroenterologist[13] working at the Middlesex Hospital, London. They compared a group of 31 patients with 'non-organic' abdominal pain with a similar number of patients with peptic ulcers or with other definite physical pathologies. Compared with the controls, the patients with non-organic pain complained of more-or-less constant pain, unrelieved by food and sometimes made worse by it. There was distension and belching, nausea but not much vomiting, and seldom any weight loss. From the psychosocial point of view in 16 of the 31, one or both parents had suffered abdominal pain, and in seven of these patients the onset of symptoms was 'closely associated' with the death of a parent. In 12 patients 'the pain seemed to be significantly related to difficulties with a spouse or a girlfriend'. Six were found to be depressed. The researchers found that their patients 'tended to be conscientious with high standards of personal behaviour'.

This study showed that significant differences could be demonstrated between those with 'organic' and 'non-organic' pain, in both symptomatology and psychosocial history, but these differences could not on their own enable anyone to exclude an organic cause for a patient's pain. It is also widely held that patients with psychogenic pain use elaborate phraseology to describe their experience but this can be a trap for the unwary.[12] Although a large number of people do undoubtedly experience pain of psychological origin, the positive recognition of psychogenic pain (that is diagnosing psychogenic pain without first having excluded physical explanations) requires considerable clinical experience of the physical conditions which might possibly be at the root of it; such a diagnosis should never be made because a patient appears nervy, uses picturesque descriptions or otherwise conforms to the stereotype of the 'neurotic'.

Where 'acute' pain is concerned — that is the kind of pain in an abdominal emergency or in the early postoperative days — the differentiation can be easier since the problem may be one of acute anxiety. The patient who almost rolls off the bed in agony can usually be soothed by a calm manner and quiet talking. If not, an intravenous injection of some sedative drug can settle the symptom in seconds. Then the doctor can try to discover what the real problem is and, incidentally, can make a physical examination in peace. The best training for recognizing psychogenic pain is a good knowledge of the varieties of presentation of physical illness.

There has been some experimental work on the identification of psychogenic pain using the evoked potentials on the electroencephalogram.[14,15] Four groups of patients were investigated: 25 'normal subjects', 18 psychiatric patients without pain (three of them had been previously diagnosed as having psychogenic pain), nine patients with pain due to carcinoma and 25 patients with psychogenic pain.

Those in the first three groups responded in essentially the same way: there was a linear correlation between the intensity of ulnar nerve stimulation and the amplitude of the evoked response on the cerebral cortex. The patients with psychogenic pain showed no such correlation, and there were greater differences between individuals. Also, they tended to produce their maximal cortical response 'at a significantly lower intensity of stimulation'.[16]

Chronic or intractable pain

These are the patients who present the real pain problems in clinical practice. 'Acute' pain is easy to treat, and anyway it is by definition self-limiting. The term 'chronic' or better 'intractable' is reserved for those patients whose pain persists despite the conventional remedies. The distinction between physical and psychogenic pain is difficult with these patients but doctors may not press investigations to begin with because they know that most people's pains go with time.

If pain continues different analgesics will be tried and there will be referral to appropriate specialists. All this can cover several months or even years so that by the time the patient has become recognized as a 'pain problem' the symptoms have become entrenched, the patient has slipped into a different life-style and subtle changes of attitude can have occurred in which the pain becomes a central issue in the person's life and all kinds of apparently unrelated matters are subsumed to it. Already at this stage powerful psychological and social factors can be seen to be operating (one of the most important of these is anticipated compensation), and it is often easy to see how a tendency on the part of the patient to slip into invalidism was fostered by delays and failure to seize the essence of the problem. Very easy to see with hindsight: very difficult at the time to pick out the potentially chronic pain patient from the large numbers presenting with painful conditions.

The presence of physical and psychological factors in varying degrees, and with the relative proportions of these changing from time to time, makes comprehension of these people and their problems especially difficult. There is an understandable tendency to treat those pains, such as nerve root pains, which seem amenable to physical treatment, and to temporize with the rest. This is not necessarily wise as the emphasis on physical methods may permit the patient to disregard various possibly distressing psychosocial issues, so that management becomes formulated in terms of finding the right drug, injection technique, or the like. Every patient who fails to respond to the initial practitioner's treatment within the expected time-scale should be subjected to a thorough psychosocial scrutiny, and only when this has been done should any of the more specialized techniques for the relief of pain be employed.

This psychosocial scrutiny can present some problems because it is hard to know what precisely to look for beyond the usual gross social disturbances or the various psychiatric syndromes. Considerable effort has gone into trying to identify specific factors which might render one person more prone to respond adversely to pain than another. One quite elaborate statistical study of 100 patients with intractable pain[8] identified a number of themes such as might be found amongst any group of chronically sick people. There have also been a number of personality-inventory studies but so far they have not been very illuminating at the practical level.[17-19]

The problem of pain is easier to comprehend with regard to the individual patient, and it can be explored in certain specific ways:
1. What is the significance of the pain for the patient?
2. Has the location of the pain any special importance?
3. Why did the pain start when it did?
4. Is it relevant that the symptom is pain rather than any other equally limiting symptom?

The significance of the pain for the patient

The simplest way into this question is to examine the effects the pain has had on the person's life: joint pains (with minimal bony changes) may have a profoundly limiting effect on someone's mobility, headaches may interfere with particular activities, pelvic pain often reduces sexual activity. The pain may also be communicating some message. For example, a 53-year-old married woman was referred by the orthopaedic surgeons as her fairly typical low back pain radiating down the right leg had not responded to conservative measures. She arrived in a wheelchair, unable to walk unaided. Six years before the present illness, she described how her second husband went out one day to buy a packet of cigarettes but never returned, and had not been heard of since. Having then to fend for herself, she found a good job, but there was a fire at the works and she was made redundant. Her next job in an engineering works was unsatisfying to her. She felt more and more isolated far from her native town, and the back symptoms gradually developed. After admission to the psychiatric unit she was soon mobilized, and in due course found more satisfying employment with a total recovery from her back symptoms. Her pain appeared to be the expression of her great need to be dependent on someone, and to have someone to care for her. At any rate this formulation was justified by events because when this need was met she began to improve.

Location of the pain

A 35-year-old mother of two teenage boys was referred to a surgeon with the complaint of pain in the left lower leg. The patient said that her foot had 'gone blue' on a number of occasions, and on one visit one inch of wasting was detected in the left thigh. The pain conformed to no familiar pattern but it persisted. Then it was noted that the patient's father had died some months before from a pulmonary embolus from a leg vein thrombosis following gastric surgery. The doctor commented on the distress with which the patient described these events, and suggested a possible association between the two sets of symptoms, but she rejected that as absurd. At psychiatric interview, it emerged that she had been very dependent upon her father, and his death had highlighted the poor relationship she had with her husband. Exploration of these issues was productive at first and her complaint of pain lessened, although coincidentally she became mildly depressed (as quite often happens when somatic symptoms disappear). Unfortunately the domestic situation proved unalterable and she never made a total recovery.

Timing of onset or exacerbation of pain

This can sometimes give a direct clue to the problem, as with a 54-year-old unmarried secretary who presented with a six-year history of pain and cramp in the right hand. It dated from the time her company moved its offices to less agreeable surroundings which also involved an arduous journey to and from work. By the time she had been seen by a psychiatrist she had had neck traction and a carpal tunnel decompression, but the pain had continued. Further inquiry revealed that she was living alone with her 86-year-old mother in a house which would be sold when the old lady died, leaving the patient with no home and no possibility of getting one. Once the pressing social problems were out in the open the pain and cramps were mentioned no more and she was able to work unimpeded by it. Her general practitioner was able to give her a certain amount of support to cope with her worrying domestic situation.

Certain pains, such as abdominal and low back pains, may have a sexual significance (as well of course as possibly being the consequence of pathology of the sex organs). Pains associated by the patient as coming from particular organs well may have a significance according to the significance that part has for the patient.

The relevance of pain

The relevance of pain, as opposed to any other symptom which from the psychological point of view could equally draw attention to the patient's distress, leads back to formulations about the meaning of pain for the individual. Most people, apart from those taking up a stance of denial, will have reflected upon this for themselves but they may be slow to talk about such things to a tough-minded doctor in a busy clinic, for their thoughts may contain all kinds of private fantasies about the pain, particularly in terms of punishment for real or imagined wrongdoing, or even for having what are regarded as wicked thoughts.

George Engel of Rochester, New York, who has made substantial contributions to knowledge of psychophysical interactions, chose a qualitative approach when trying to discover something about the meaning of pain for individual patients.[20] He listed some of the meanings which he felt pain had for his patients, in addition to its function as a warning mechanism. In infancy pain leads to crying which in turn leads to comforting by the mother, and so in adult life the symptom of pain may be associated with a need to be comforted. Also in childhood pain may be linked with punishment (which is what *poena,* the Latin origin of the word, means). Pain early on becomes associated with agression through the infliction of pain upon others, but in psychological language this kind of aggression can be turned against the self, building up bodily tensions which may lead to pain. Also guilt on account of these aggressive feelings may manifest itself as pain. Engel concludes:

> Some of these individuals are chronically depressive, pessimistic and gloomy people whose guilty, self-deprecating attitudes are readily apparent from the moment they walk into your office. They seem to have had no joy or enthusiasm for life ... They drift into situations or submit to relationships in which they are hurt, beaten, defeated, humiliated and ... at the same time they conspicuously fail to exploit situations which should lead to successes ...

Neither this qualitative study nor the quantitative studies described earlier leads to the elaboration of any clear general principles concerning intractable pain although a number of insights are offered. It still remains to be established whether pain has a special significance in its own right or whether it is merely another manifestation of incapacity through a chronic condition such as lameness or breathlessness. Nevertheless, I find Engel's views interesting although they are difficult to utilize in practice.

Investigation into these specific aspects of the pain experience should come at the end of a general psychosocial inquiry. When dealing with such a powerful symptom as pain it is important to keep the personal discussion separate otherwise the conversation always returns to the topic of pain. A non-medical interviewer has an advantage here as he can ignore clinical details as being outside his competence. In this psychosocial inquiry particular note will be taken of the timing of major events. The interviewer should have a detailed chronology of the pain beforehand, and coincidences can be quietly noted as he goes along, but they should not be pointed out to the patient until he is ready to consider them, otherwise such associations will be rejected out of hand, and the interviewer may be rejected also.

The relevance of the association between, say, the onset of pain and a bereavement becomes apparent through the emotion expressed or through the obvious importance of the life-event, but most of all the relevance is established by being able to use such information to enable the patient to make clinical progress.

Pain clinics

Neurosurgeons and individual anaesthetists have for years taken an interest in pain relief, but the mass of new techniques has led to the introduction of specialized clinics where a great deal of expertise can be deployed.[7] They can also provide interesting clinical opportunities for anaesthetists and physiologists. Unfortunately perhaps, these people are entering clinical practice at a peculiarly difficult point. Somatic symptoms of possible psychological origin are easy enough to recognize but difficult to eliminate. Furthermore, the interaction of physical and psychosocial factors requires an approach which can abide with the paradoxes of human behaviour, and which is not likely to come easily to the kind of mind which is at its best when grappling with the mechanical problems inherent in direct action against nerve roots and the like.

There is a danger that pain clinics will become technical wonder houses with longer needles being aimed with ever-increasing accuracy, and all the patients' problems being interpreted in terms of physical processes. Psychiatrists and social workers may be welcomed into this environment if they look as if they can remove the awkward cases who fail to respond as expected to the treatments offered, but what is really needed is partnership. A requirement of such partnership is that the psychiatrists and social workers grapple with the mechanical principles of pain relief so that they can understand what their colleagues are doing, and also be more supportive and acceptable to their patients. Conversely, the staff in pain clinics will have to acquire an understanding of the conceptual framework within which the psychiatrists and social workers function. This does not mean learning about different varieties of mental disorder but rather about principles of psychological development, interpersonal relationships, responses to stress, and so on, such as can be found in D. Russell Davis's book *An Introduction to Psychopathology*.[21] The two kinds of clinical workers – the technical and the psychosocial – function and conceptualize in such totally different ways that a real effort has to be made if each is to understand the principles and metaphor of the other. In this kind of coming together the technological worker always has the harder task.

Summary

Pain cannot be experienced except by a conscious subject, and the experience can be drastically modified (or eliminated altogether) by cultural, psychological and other factors. A physical lesion is not a pre-requisite for pain, and psychogenic pain is common in all branches of medical practice. Problems of chronic or intractable pain usually involve a complex of physical and psychological factors, and understanding of the individual patient involves understanding the meaning of the pain for that person. Pain clinics can concentrate expertise, but there should be a partnership with the psychosocial workers and not an exclusive concern with the technical aspects of pain relief.

9. Aftermath of Treatment

Life may be preserved but at a price. The body may not function as it used to, the patient may no longer feel acceptable as an ordinary member of society or as a sexual partner, and the perception of the self — the self-image — may have changed or even become unrecognizable.

Amputation

When a limb is lost just about every activity has to be re-learned at least in some degree. The physical loss is visible to all: the psychological loss generally has to be contained. There is an intense preoccupation with what has been lost, emotions equivalent to mourning, but it is hard to mourn the loss of a limb openly because there are no conventions and rituals connected with its disposal, and it is not something that people are expected to grieve over anyway.

Phases of grief may be observed among amputees similar to those endured by bereaved people.[1,2] At first there is a kind of *numbness* or disbelief, then a period of *pining*, leading on to *depression* in some degree, and most important the phase of *reorganization* or readjustment in which the patient is forced 'to give up one view of his world and himself in it and to replace it with another'.

Post-amputation pain at first sight seems such an obviously physical condition with scar tissue (presumably) irritating the cut ends of the nerves that the patient's experience can easily be overlooked. Once the focus of interest shifts from

100

the stump to the person a variety of psychosocial issues may be discovered which can account for slow recovery and persistent pain.[3] Some of the factors which can be used with reasonable reliability to predict which patients will be having 'persistent pain' 13 months after amputation are:

> some pain in the phantom at three weeks after amputation, a high score on a scale measuring 'compulsive self-reliance' [summed up in the sentiment: 'there are two kinds of people in the world, the weak and the strong'] and amputation which follows an illness of more than one year's duration[4]

Loss of uterus

The uterus has generally done all the work it is going to do by the time it becomes an object of interest to the gynaecological surgeon. To the rationalist it is by then a piece of redundant tissue which henceforth can only cause trouble. It can be removed in twenty minutes, the woman will lose her symptoms and also the source of a substantial risk of cancer. Therefore large numbers of women in their thirties and forties who have irregular bleeding, or practically any intractable symptom referable to the pelvis, end up losing their womb. Not many, it seems, are asked by their busy male gynaecologists what they feel about their womb, and if it has any special significance for them with regard to their sense of feminity, but the follow-up of women after hysterectomy shows a good deal of distress. Women are more likely to become depressed or to develop other psychological symptoms after hysterectomy than after other operations of comparable mechanical severity (such as cholecystectomy), and these symptoms are most likely, and referral to psychiatrists more than twice as common, when no significant physical pathology is found at operation.[5-8] Thus it would seem that where disorders of uterine function are concerned (as opposed to structural lesions) some element in the origin of the disorder is not being dealt with by removing the uterus.

Loss of a breast

A breast matters to a woman. Male surgeons might remember

this better if it was the penis that was to be removed, and if the defect would somehow be clearly visible to the public gaze unless careful restorative measures were taken.

Breast surgery is discussed so much by surgeons that the breast itself loses sexual significance. Indeed, the emotional detachment with which a surgeon contemplates the possibly diseased breast in a clinic can lead him to deny that it possesses any significance at all except in terms of abnormal and potentially dangerous tissue. The management of breast lumps is such a well practised routine that surgeons will often adopt a breezy, confident attitude in terms of 'We'll have that off in no time' or 'It's no more use to you anyway'. An atmosphere of 'jollying along' and busyness can inhibit women who usually have the most painful anxieties about their survival and their future as sexual beings, and a number of studies have shown that there is more distress and a greater number of problems in rehabilitation than surgeons seem to realize.[9-13]

Imagine the woman who after the operation feels for her breast. The student nurse knows nothing. The junior doctor talks about microscopic examination. The surgeon is reassuring, but of course the only reassurance worth having cannot be given by anyone.

Radiotherapy is difficult. It is a reasonable extra precaution, but many patients assume it is only for the hopeless cases. It can also be frightening, and some modern units have a science fiction quality about them. Preoperative explanation that radiotherapy is part of the overall plan (if it is) can reduce anxiety.

Most important of all, the woman has to come to terms with the new topography of her body. She is asymmetrical, or 'misshapen', 'peculiar', 'mutilated' or 'lopsided'. It is difficult for her to look at herself in a mirror, and she turns away from her husband when she undresses. She feels perhaps that no man would want a woman like that.

The breast to be sacrificed may have fulfilled its function abundantly, as witnessed by the happy family around the woman, or it may be a bitter sacrifice which will preclude that fulfillment for ever. Where there is a husband, he should be involved at every stage, unless the woman has some substantial reasons for excluding him. The husband may have difficulty in accepting his wife once she is no longer an intact sex object, more difficulty perhaps in coping with his side of the problem than the wife has with hers. The surgical crisis may bring them closer together, but equally it may reopen unresolved conflicts and blow the marriage apart. Divorce after breast surgery is not uncommon.

The children will wonder what has happened to mother. Young ones will see it in terms of mother's absence and reduced energy. Older children will be able to comprehend the threat to the family, and teenage girls can relate mother's experience to themselves. It is better for children to suffer whatever shock there may be in seeing their mother's bony chest than for them to develop fantasies which are likely to be worse than the reality.

The teenage daughter now may become the only complete woman in the home. If the woman becomes 'a bird with broken wings' she may feel, and with justification perhaps, that her husband now treats his young daughter as he used to treat his wife. Daughter and mother can get into a conflict (and this happens after hysterectomies also) which neither comprehends.

Resumption of sexual life

The first private encounter between husband and wife after returning home is important. The couple have got to recognize one another anew. If the husband has been closely involved from the start he will have been changed by his experiences, and that may make it easier for them both to see the return home in terms of a new beginning. Love-making may be painful and awkward at first because of the chest scars. She may, for a while at any rate, want to avoid love-making. An appreciable number of women develop a distaste for sex after mastectomy despite a considerate and interested partner. Most women will see a mastectomy as marking the end of their fertile life (although this is not inevitable), and may develop an aversion to intercourse after any measure which will (or they think will) render them sterile. For them sex for pleasure alone may bring various sexual conflicts to the surface. Another group will avoid sex because of their feelings of self-debasement, that they are no longer truly feminine, and that no man could really want them however much the man might demonstrate his interest. This is part of the inevitable reaction to the loss, part of a mourning process in which the subject is personifying her sense of incompleteness. Because of the feelings of shame involved, these sentiments are not likely to be offered to male surgeons in hospital clinics but they are expressed in sympathetic and unhurried interviews, as the surveys show. Occasionally, when a woman becomes depressed after the removal of a breast, the feelings pour out: passionate insistence of unworthiness because all her feelings of self-respect and sexual identity have become focussed on the lost breast, anger against the surgeons for real or imagined misdeeds, anger against her husband whom she may accuse of taking up with other women.

Breast prosthesis

The best breast prosthesis costs a fraction of the cost of accommodating a patient for one day in a large hospital but attending to the fine details of an artifical breast does not come easily to many surgeons. It may be that to them the breast is an erotic object and they can only treat it as such or, because of their medical training, as an object of clinical interest. Their own emotional immaturity may prevent them from empathizing with the woman's point of view. Also, many surgeons hold on to a generally tough-minded attitude to any aspect of surgery which relates to appearance, as though all that really matters is function. It is as if there were older, rougher boys at school still looking over their shoulders ready to call them 'sissy' if they showed too much concern for cosmetic effect. This tendency applies to all scars wherever they may be, even on the face.

It is debatable when the question of prostheses should be introduced. It could be discussed with a specialist fitter before even coming into hospital with the happy possibility that it would not be needed, but every patient who loses a breast should have something to wear in its place when she leaves hospital, and then a prosthesis of the best available quality can be arranged at leisure.

Artificial openings

It has been estimated that in the United States there are over one million people with artifical openings, or stomas, of various kinds, and that this number will double in the 1980s.[14] The great majority will be colostomies and ileostomies, but an increasing number of urinary conduits are also being performed.

Most people with permanent stomas manage impressively well and have coped successfully with a difficult adaptation. However, few manage this without a good deal of anguish, particularly in the early stages, about how other people are going to react to them, and how their friends and workmates will respond if the ever-feared spillage occurs. This theme crops up repeatedly in the accounts of the progress of stoma patients.[14-19]

Someone coming to colostomy following surgery for cancer of the large bowel may only have a relatively short history of indisposition and so be in basically good health. Anyone having an ileostomy for ulcerative colitis or Crohn's disease is liable either to be, or to have been, seriously debilitated or toxic. The patient having an ileal conduit formed may have suffered from uncontrollable incontinence or else will have serious disease of the lower urinary tract. These are, of course, technically and physiologically very different entities, but from the psychosocial point of view many aspects of artificial openings can be considered together, though this account is based on experiences with colostomies and ileostomies.

Psychological factors are regarded as being of importance in the aetiology and in influencing the clinical course of ulcerative colitis[20,21] and Crohn's disease,[22,23] but these factors will not necessarily impede the postoperative course and adjustment, possibly quite the reverse.

The first critical moment comes when the patient catches

his initial glimpse of the opening on his abdominal wall. The feelings and facial expression of the nurse or doctor removing the dressings will be all-important. It will be like toilet training all over again for the patient: messes and admonitions perhaps, then more messes which always seem to be beyond the patient's control and which can come just after the previous dressing has been completed. The patient is almost forced into a regressive state because of his initial physical helplessness, plus another kind of infantile behaviour in the form of lack of sphincter control. Even when there is no mess there can be smell, and the noise of escaping gas which also smells. It is difficult for the nurse to react enthusiastically to a newly formed stoma, but the surgeon can. He can allow himself to reveal his pride and satisfaction at a well formed spout or loop, and can let the patient into some of the technicalities.

The first view the spouse has of the stoma also matters. Wives, it seems, are often happy to irrigate and generally look after the stomas of their husbands, but women prefer to get other women to help them. A certain amount of grief will be experienced for what has been lost, but the loss of anus, although more poignant than most might suppose, is not the primary concern, as it may be after amputation or mastectomy: the emphasis is more on the opening which has been gained. For a while there may be sensations of a phantom rectum,[24] and a varying degree of depression. On the other hand, when the stoma is an ileostomy there may be such a rapid recovery of physical well-being that the early stages will be psychologically uneventful.

Going out in public involves a good deal of anxiety about spillage, noises and smells, as any doctor would realize if he went shopping by bus with a plastic bag of liquid faeces strapped to his abdomen. No matter how good appliances become there will always be an element of anxiety, and it can easily become the focus for other unrelated anxieties in the patient's life and lead to a consequent limitation of mobility. For a good many there will be a reduction in social and other activities but this will apply mainly to the older age groups with colostomies who have had operations for cancer. Among the over-65s, a much higher than expected frequency of social isolation is reported by people with colostomies, especially by women from lower social classes.[25]

For the younger age groups with ileostomies, mainly done for inflammatory disease, anything seems possible — skiing, horse riding, bicycling, dancing, camping, gliding, and even under-water swimming. Only golf seems to present a problem because twisting the trunk tends to loosen the appliance.[26]

Sexual acceptance is more complicated as there can be physical impairment resulting from the operation and mechanical and aesthetic problems. This applies mainly to those in the older age groups. Among younger patients the majority, with patience and a little ingenuity in coping with the appliance, manage to enjoy a full sex life, and this is testified by the large number of women with ileostomies who go through straightforward pregnancies and the delivery of healthy babies.[18]

When there has been an extensive scar, and perhaps post-operative wound infection and peristomal skin excoriation, the abdomen can look a mess. This can do such damage to people's sense of acceptability that they may isolate themselves and become depressed, and adopt the almost unshakeable opinion that no one could possibly want them. I have known one girl with an ileostomy and a badly puckered abdominal scar who rebuffed a genuinely interested boy on the grounds that he could not sincerely be fond of anybody with an abdomen like hers.

Homosexual men who have an anal resection and a stoma are in a special predicament. In a series of 70 men having anorectal excisions and colostomies for cancer two were homosexual,[25] which is about what would be expected if it is true that 5% of the male population is homosexual. Their plight must be taken seriously, and they would be likely to benefit from the help of those accustomed to advise on psychosexual problems.

Irrigation of the colostomy can sometimes receive excessive attention, and some bad habits have been recorded, including the use of many gallons of water, and hours taken to obtain a 'crystal clear return'.[17] What is a mechanical procedure for the staff may have some emotional significance for the patient, and attempts at impossible levels of cleanliness may represent the patient's attempts to compensate for supposed feelings of being unclean.

Stomas can also become objects of sexual interest, like any other orifice. Indeed, it has been suggested that the junction of skin and mucuous membrane, whether occurring naturally or artificially, has when stimulated 'an inherent capacity for arousing feeling and emotion'.[27]

Helping the stoma patient

The stoma patient in most Western countries is well endowed with potential sources of support, though ileostomy patients seem to have more than colostomy patients. There is the surgeon, the general practitioner, specialist stoma therapist, associations of stoma patients, and community nursing and social services.

The surgeon, nursing sister, stoma therapist, patient and spouse (if any) can meet before the operation to discuss appliances and the exact siting for the stoma. Patients have views about what they feel they can and cannot manage, and elderly and partially sighted patients can have special problems. Some have preferences for transparent, and others for opaque appliances.

It is often possible through the stoma associations to arrange for someone matching the future stoma patient to come and visit preoperatively. The right people, who have adapted well to stoma life (and have not gone overboard with enthusiasm), are liable to be in great demand for this delicate task, and they can be a great help, but this should augment rather than replace the opportunity for frank and relaxed discussion with professional helpers.

The surgeon who fashions a stoma has a patient for life whom he will see personally, and not delegate to the latest junior on his team. Every patient should leave hospital fully briefed about stoma care and with all necessary spare parts. The stoma therapist will generally raise the question of sexual adjustment, which will be a matter of intense concern to most patients, because so few patients will feel able to raise the matter themselves.

Iatrogenic sexual dysfunction

Hernia repair

It often makes for a better repair of a recurrent inguinal hernia in an elderly man to remove the testis and spermatic cord. Looking at the shrivelled organs as one paints and towels up before operation it is so easy to say: 'He won't be needing it now' — whatever 'it' might be. I have said this myself in the past on such occasions, but, I must now confess, without any real understanding of what I was saying, and certainly without any awareness of the elderly patient as a sexual being who might value his organs as much as I do mine.

The question of removal of the testis should be discussed with the elderly man with the same gravity as if he was 25, instead of treating him as though he already was on some masculine scrap-heap. It is, of course, the surgeon's first responsibility to do a good job of repair, but a plastic testis is simple to install, and may give valuable support for a diminishing masculine self-image.

Prostate

Despite the widespread occurrence of prostatic enlargement, and the fact that it explicitly involves the sexual organs, I know of only two studies published in the last ten years which consider the effect of prostatic surgery on sexual function. In one of the studies[28] 67% of 102 men were potent before operation (which meant that they had the desire for sexual intercourse, the ability to attain an erection, and to ejaculate), and 84% of these retained their potency postoperatively. In the other survey[29] of 94 men undergoing suprapubic or transurethral prostatectomy for benign enlargement, 80% of those aged 60 or less retained their potency, and 33% of those aged 61 to 80. Five of their series said their sexual performance had improved following operation.

Although a number of patients will find retrograde ejaculation into the bladder distressing, the outcome of prostatic surgery for benign enlargement from the point of view of sexual performance is good. Patients with a willing and physically able partner, and with the benefit of more refined surgical techniques, need not feel that prostatectomy heralds the onset of decrepit old age. On the other hand, certain patients may welcome the excuse for avoiding sexual demands which they had for some time been finding hard to meet.

Rectum

There is no general agreement about the incidence of failure of erection or ejaculation following damage to the pelvic nerve supply during dissection around the rectum in the male during operations for cancer.[25,30] This is probably due to the fact that the debilitating effect of surgery, and the depression associated with having cancer and a colostomy as well, will hasten the reduction of sexual activity which can be expected amongst these patients, many of whom are over 60. Nevertheless, mechanical damage does occur but the best index of this may be from the incidence of urinary disturbance[31] (as the bladder has the same nerve supply as the genitalia) where the effects of ageing and the aesthetic and emotional influences will be less important.

After operations for inflammatory disease of the rectum the likelihoood of damage to sympathetic and parasympathetic nerve supply to the sexual organs is less than after operations for cancer.[26,32,33] Among the small proportion of patients who have lost the ability to attain erection and to ejaculate, the majority in the surveys were over 50, which suggests that psychological factors and the processes of ageing might also be involved as these older patients were not indicated as having extensive disease requiring extra drastic dissection. On the other hand, the differential loss of the power of erection or ejaculation does point more to mechanical damage.

Abdominal aorta

Around one-third to two-thirds of patients presenting with

atherosclerotic disease of the abdominal aorta have some impairment of erection[34,35,36] This may be due to the disease itself or to associated diabetes. After clearing out of the blocked arteries a few with existing sexual potency may lose it through damage to the sympathetic nerves, but others again may recover their potency especially when by careful dissection the sympathetic nerves have been left intact.[36]

Mechanical problems after gynaecological surgery

Most medical students and junior doctors make a brief excursion into gynaecological surgery by performing an *episiotomy* or at any rate by stitching up after one has been done. The experience of 237 Australian women three months after delivery suggests that this excursion should perhaps be more of a guided tour. They had all had a mediolateral episiotomy, and 39% of them had suffered painful intercourse, which remained severe and persistent in 6%.[37]

After the *Wertheim hysterectomy* for carcinoma (the upper one-third of the vagina is removed and there is a wider excision of tissue within the pelvis), considerable difficulties may be experienced. A cooperative partner is needed to assist in stretching the vagina by gentle intercourse which should commence about three months after operation.[38]

Where radiotherapy is used as the sole or partial treatment of cervical carcinoma severe vaginal fibrosis can be expected, leading to narrowing, and loss of the response of lubrication due to fibrosis of the perivaginal venous plexuses. In a series from New York City,[39] 22 of 28 patients having cervical cancer treated by radiotherapy alone suffered changes in sexual function, and 22 (more or less but not entirely the same group as above) developed 'narrowing or obliteration of at least two-thirds of the vagina'. By contrast, of the 32 patients treated by surgery alone, two described adverse changes in sexual function and three were found to have vaginal narrowing. Where radiotherapy and surgery were combined, five out of 15 had some sexual dysfunction, and nine had vaginal narrowing.

Since patients are not asked routinely about their sexual function it is difficult for doctors to evaluate its importance in planning treatment, but clearly if five-year survival rates following surgery alone and radiotherapy alone are similar, the question of sexual activity is important. However, I do not know whether this is the kind of decision that patients could reasonably be expected to make amid all the distress at having a diagnosis of malignancy. It is an area where we are all rather ignorant but we will learn as we come to discuss these matters more freely with our patients. The gastric surgeon, Lord Moynihan, is reputed to have said 'we must not give up living in order to live'.

About 20% of patients undergoing *repair operations for uterine prolapse* may have severe difficulties in sexual relations after operation.[40] These may be due to deliberate tightening which was judged an inevitable price to pay for urinary continence, to lack of judgement on the part of the surgeon, or to lack of a partner to keep at bay (by coitus) the processes of senile or postoperative contracture. The risk of such problems is greatest after posterior repair (colpoperineorrhaphy).

Haemodialysis and transplantation

Chronic renal failure is associated with a reduction in sexual activity; haemodialysis and transplantation reduce it further. This was the conclusion of a nationwide postal questionnaire survey of patients in the United States who had undergone haemodialysis and/or transplantation.[41] Not the best way of gathering information about such private matters, but there were before-and-after comparisons, and it is one way of getting large numbers of respondents — 345 men and 174 women.

Some 48% of the men and 26% of the women reported the appearance of or worsening of sexual problems (inadequate erection and/or 'decrease in sexual drive') with the progress of uraemia before starting on haemodialysis. Once haemodialysis was started, out of the original group 8% of the men and 6% of the women experienced an improvement of sexual function, but 35% of the men and 25% of the women experienced a worsening. These findings are in line with smaller studies based on personal interview.[42,43] Despite the deterioration in sex life there is an improvement in general health which would make the deterioration in sex life seem rather paradoxical. With regard to *transplantation,* the postal survey does not suggest it leads to a better sex life than haemodialysis as far as men are concerned. The women, however, are not so adversely affected as the men.

Drugs

Various drugs which block neural conduction can inhibit sexual responses, most notably hexamethonium which blocks parasympathetic and sympathetic transmissions, and so erection and ejaculation respectively are abolished. Any sedative drug is liable to damp down responses to the level where a man is impotent, and a high level of anxiety can itself inhibit the ability to attain an erection, so drug treatment for anxiety states can be problematical from the point of view of improving sexual performance. Phenothiazines and benzodiazepines are the most important drugs in this connection, and also the tricyclic antidepressants by their anticholinergic action.[44]

Summary

Amputation, loss of uterus or breast, colostomy and ileostomy can all involve psychological and psychosexual problems in addition to the physical processes of recuperation. Certain interventions such as drug treatments, hernia repair, surgery to the prostate, rectum, abdominal aorta and gynaecological organs, and also haemodialysis and kidney transplantation are commonly followed by physical impairments to sexual functioning.

10. Beyond Cure

All the chapters so far have dealt one way or another with illness. The doctor is healthy, he may never experience illness or incapacity, but he certainly will die. Doctors share death with their patients, and a dying doctor is no different from any other dying person. Death therefore could represent a common ground where all the resistances and peculiarities of doctors could finally be resolved, and where the doctor and patient could meet on more equal terms in the recognition that the patient was simply making *his* final journey slightly before the doctor.

Yet it is this very fact that death is something common to doctor and patient which may be the crucial reason why doctors are so helpless in the face of death, why they act so defensively, or even deny its reality at all. The care of the dying is sadly neglected when compared with facilities available for the cure of those with dramatic illnesses, but the provision of care is still effectively determined by the collective will of doctors, and doctors collectively are not interested in the dying.

I believe this lack of active concern can be understood by looking into the person of the doctor, and any doctor who feels uneasy in his contact with dying people and wants to do better by them will do well to look within himself. No one can care for dying people who has not already come to terms with his own mortality.

114

Talking to people with incurable illnesses

Practically everybody, whether they work in the health industry or not, has views about how much people should or should not know about their final illnesses. I have never met anyone who felt the issue was unimportant. This passionate concern is never quite convincing because it is not real concern for the dying person but rather concern for the peace of mind of the healthy. And how often do these healthy people ask the dying what they feel about dying?

Some years ago when cancer education was much in people's minds, a number of surveys were carried out concerning 'what to tell the patient'. They emphasize the differing attitudes of doctors and patients.

Doctors' views

In an inquiry into the habits of 444 medical specialists and general practitioners in Philadelphia, 69% 'never' told or 'usually' did not tell patients that they had cancer, although they often felt that a responsible member of the family should be told.[1]

In another study, out of 219 doctors on the staff of one teaching hospital in Chicago, around 88% had a policy 'not to tell', and there were no significant differences according to specialty, age or experience. The reasons for not telling were given not in terms of 'cool scientific judgement' but as a rigidly held 'personal conviction'. 'Highly charged and emotional terms and vivid expressions were the rule, indicating the intensity and nature of the feelings present.' Questionnaires were used in addition to personal interviews but, as the author said, it was 'not necessary to read the words on the questionnaires. Heavy underlining and a peppering of exclamation points [told] the story'. 77% of the respondents said that 'clinical experience' was the principal determining factor in their attitudes, and they cited examples of despondency and suicide, but when pressed only 14% had had any direct experience of a policy with regard to telling or not telling which was different from their current one. When the author probed further by asking what the policy of the respondents was towards the results of research in general into what to tell patients with cancer, 16% 'indicated that their policy would not be swayed by research'. Another 29% were uncertain whether or not they would accept the findings of any such research, while 10% felt 'that research in this area should not be done at all'. All this was from doctors at a teaching hospital 'who read assiduously and themselves conduct research'. By contrast, nearly 60% felt that they would want to be told if they had cancer. 'I am one of those who could take it' or 'I have responsibilities' were usual explanations.[2]

Another way of avoiding the painful realities of cancer is not to diagnose it, and this tendency of doctors was discussed in Chapter 5, especially the occasions when doctors are slow to recognize or to admit the existence of cancer in themselves or in their medical colleagues.

Patients' views

The great majority of patients want to be told the truth about themselves. In Minneapolis 89% of a group of 100 cancer patients with operable or inoperable lesions 'preferred knowing their condition' and 73% of the group thought that all people should be told their diagnosis. In a group of 100 patients at the same hospital without cancer, 82% said they would want to be told if they developed cancer, and so did 98% of 740 people attending a cancer detection centre.[3]

A study some years later from the same centre reported 87% of 298 patients who had survived five to twenty years after cancer treatment knew their diagnosis and 93% of these stated that knowing the diagnosis had been a 'distinct advantage'. A group of 92 patients with advanced malignancies were then asked the same questions, and of the 86 who knew their diagnosis, 87% also said the information had been an advantage.[4] The reasons given for wanting to know are interesting (see the table on p. 117).

In Manchester, as part of a cancer education programme, a series of 231 men and women with cancers thought to be

	Treated cases (%) (n = 253)	Advanced cases (%) (n = 77)
Help in understanding illness	67	60
Help in planning follow-up medical care	66	48
Making for peace of mind	42	55
Decrease in worry about health	32	18
Planning religious matters	30	17
Planning own future	26	29
Planning family future	26	21
Planning financial matters	26	21

treatable were told their diagnosis routinely 'quite un-
emotionally and casually'. Between a week and a month later
they were asked their reactions to receiving this information.
66% 'approved' of having been told, 7% 'disapproved' of
having been told, while 19% denied they had been told they
had cancer. The remainder gave inconclusive replies. Forty-
one of these patients were seen between one and two and a
half years later, and the great majority of them had not
changed their views.[5]

Looking round a surgical ward I sometimes wonder,
behind all the mis-communication and secrecy, just what the
patients really know about the nature of their illnesses. Two
investigators in Finland interviewed 100 men and women
with common cancers to try and answer this question.[6]
Forty of the patients were told the diagnosis explicitly by
their doctors. The majority were satisfied with the way they
had been told although five denied having been told the
diagnosis at all. Another 29 had asked their doctors for the
diagnosis and these turned out to be more satisfied on the
whole than those who had had the information given them
unasked for. 24 did not ask and were not told. Altogether
two-thirds knew their diagnosis, and the majority of these
developed symptoms: 'tenseness, depression, fear of death,
anxiety, aggressiveness' etc. but none expressed suicidal
thoughts. If there was any criticism of being told or of the
way they were told, a number felt the subject might have
been introduced more gradually, and that hope should never
be destroyed.

Discrepancy between doctors' views and patients' views

From the surveys cited and also from numerous personal accounts it seems that the great majority of patients want to know what is the matter with them but, in Britain at any rate, the doctors do not want to tell them. This reticence on the part of doctors is declining, and in many countries doctors are obliged to reveal the diagnosis. That is, they are obliged to state the bald facts. Whether they feel able to do more than that is quite another matter. There is not much difference in the quality of personal support a patient is getting from the doctor whether he says 'It's just a little cyst, we'll have it out next week', or 'I'm afraid the lump is malignant, we'll operate next week'. The same personal defensiveness can remain, however explicit the doctor may be; indeed bluntness of speech is just one way the doctor can make patients keep their distance.

The differing views of doctors and patients towards incurable illness are not part of a wholesome conflict but of a situation where doctors are all-powerful and the patients are helpless. The doctors are simply imposing their views and feelings on vulnerable and frightened patients who are usually too distressed and too bewildered by their surroundings to stand up for themselves, and who are anyway seldom in one place long enough to understand how the system works and so how to make their views felt. The doctors, on the other hand, are on their home ground doing their routine work with no obvious extra emotional burden to bear. What attitudes then does the doctor have which can lead to such behaviour?

I do not believe that I have a right to withhold from someone the knowledge that he has a fatal disease. I believe that each person has a right to know his fate. If that person cannot handle such painful truth then psychological defence mechanisms may come into play which will dull the reality or suppress it altogether either permanently or else until the person is ready to assimilate the sad reality. But I do not feel that doctors have any right at all to deny people the chance of meeting their fate and of the possibility of that psychological or spiritual development that many people achieve when in the full awareness that their lives are drawing to a close.

Doctor's perception of his role

The whole medical education machine is directed towards curing diseases. Cures (not prevention) get the professional kudos and public acclaim: they also get the money for new departments, better equipment and bigger research projects. Few medical schools have any teaching about caring for the sick as opposed to curing the sick, and the few that do have some instruction about caring cannot put it across with the same authority and excitement as can the advocate of a new wonder drug or the enthusiastic developer of a new surgical operation. Apart from anything else, caring simply does not have the same appeal for young medical students.

Medical teaching is cure-oriented and takes place in hospital. When an incurable patient is encountered on a teaching ward round it is an embarrassment. 'What is this patient doing here?' demands the senior specialist. The message to the students is that incurable patients are not their business. Students are distressed by such behaviour but they are caught in a conflict between their own instincts and the desire to adopt the values of their teachers which they feel dimly must be part of being a good doctor, at least if the prestige jobs are going to be pursued.

The incurable patient threatens the whole cure-oriented machine, and so must either be disregarded or else the doctor's perception of his role must change. Ivan Illich has called dying 'the ultimate form of consumer resistance'.[7,8]

Doctors and death

Doctors are in the death business. In this they keep company with funeral directors, soldiers, priests, policemen, lawyers, life assurance workers, and others who work against a background of death. Death is either the explicit basis of their work or else it is there by implication, but for all it has a particular significance which will vary from group to group. Some will be accepting of death, some will be seeking it or causing it, others will be busy fighting it off. Doctors are engaged in fighting it. For their efforts they are rewarded well and admired by the communities in which they work, but are they possibly also conducting a private battle with their own anxieties about death which conceivably might have a part to play in their decision to become part of the medical profession in the first place? By becoming part of the machine which fights death might they manage to keep their own anxieties about death at bay? By fighting death it is possible to deny its reality. In fact the idea of death itself can be done away with and replaced by illnesses or pathological states. No one should just be allowed to die, as bodily processes fail they can be stimulated artificially or the function can be taken over by a machine. The outcome is not 'death' as traditionally understood, but a medical state such as 'failed cardiac resuscitation' or 'flat trace on the EEG'. This is the 'medicalization of death' to quote Illich again.[7,8]

Whatever anxieties a doctor may or may not have regarding death, he certainly meets it frequently. When he is young and freshly qualified he may find himself working in a surgical ward with perhaps six or eight dying patients. How can he cope with them and give them the kind of support they require? Even to sit and listen to their fears of dying (assuming the subject had been opened up at all) would place an intolerable emotional burden on him. In his mid-twenties he is expansive and forward-looking, keen to start real living after all the years of study, and not really at a point in life to help someone on their way out of it. Also, he finds all of a sudden that he has been given no guidance in how to cope with those who cannot be cured. The obvious fact that all patients will eventually die and that doctors are always expected to be involved at such times has not been acknowledged in medical teaching.

The young doctor can be forgiven if, in the absence of any help from his seniors, he allows defences to go up with regard to the incurable. As he gets older and reaches the point where he can perceive his own life having an end as well as a beginning, he may find that he can live with the conscious realization of the fact of death and his own mortality, and so become better able to accept the mortality of others. On the other hand the defences may become permanent and suppressed from consciousness, so that the dying patient who received such warm support in the past when his ailments were curable now turns to the doctor for help in his hour of ultimate trial and finds only the shell of a person.

Doctors and the dying

Proficiency in most branches of medicine involves acquiring information or developing practical skills. The day-to-day management of dying patients involves certain expertise, and a number of valuable guides are available from Cicely Saunders[9,10] and others.[11-15] However, the dying person can only make use of medical technology to a limited extent, and any doctor working exclusively in the conventional medical 'curing' ethos will fail to meet that person's needs. Indeed, such doctors can become intruders.

The doctor will be able to support people who are dying only if he has come to terms with certain aspects of his own being. He must accept fully that the person is beyond cure and that this state does not necessarily carry any implications of failure on his part. The doctor should assume that he has a personal need to effect cures, and so when the patient does not oblige by getting better he may be liable to feel some sense of affront, and even to feel angry and rejecting towards any patient who fails to cooperate by failing to recover.

If I operate upon someone whose condition then deteriorates from the day after the operation, I will feel bad. The condition may have been hopeless from the outset or I may have made an error of judgment: in either case the person would have been more comfortable if no operation had been performed. My feelings, whether or not they contain an element of guilt, do not make it easy for me to sit at the bedside and accept calmly that the person is beyond the expertise of doctors. Because of my training and because of what I think the patients, and of course the hospital staff, expect of me, I will feel obliged to take some action. As long as I am doing something medical, honour is satisfied and most patients and their relatives are satisfied also. But the reality of dying can be denied by medical activity.

A doctor caring for the dying has to be able to acknowledge his feelings. Cures can be effected by intellectual processes alone; caring requires that one person feels for another. Many doctors have difficulty with their feeling (nurses do also), and as a result the whole round of interaction with patients is formalized and centred around the business of diagnosis and treatment. The intellectually minded doctor is likely to feel acutely uncomfortable face to face with someone who is dying. He will feel helpless because his intellectual faculties will not help him to respond to the needs of the situation, so he may be tempted to 'do' something or else simply to retreat on the grounds of urgent business somewhere else. And the patient may not be sorry to see him go.

Only when the doctor can learn to relate through his feelings will he be of any help, but to do this he must *allow* himself to feel. I was qualified a long time before I could shed tears in front of a patient. The prospect would have been unthinkable early on in my professional life, and would have been equated by me with evidence of incompetence, but of course the reality is quite the opposite. By revealing feeling – be it by tears, or warmth, or certain kinds of anger – you become credible as a person, and that is what matters more than anything with the dying. The professional expertise is assumed: tears can show that you really care.

The discomfort and embarrassment at facing a dying person goes when a direct feeling relationship is established and the need to 'do' something is left behind. In other words, the twentieth century doctor will be able to support dying people perfectly well if he just can forget that he is a twentieth century doctor and try to act like an ordinary human being.

It will never be easy emotionally to work closely with dying people. Some will have a religious faith which motivates work with the dying, and is a powerful sustaining factor. All staff should have an opportunity to participate in group discussions where anxieties and negative emotions can be expressed freely, and these have been shown to be helpful to young doctors working on cancer units and have enabled them to become more effective in caring for their dying patients.[16]

Dying well

I have been connected with many 'bad' deaths. Throughout my surgical years death was a frequent consequence of surgical illness or of the surgery itself. For me this was especially so in cardiovascular surgery, neurosurgery, and when dealing with those shot-up in the terrorism in Cyprus. My recollections are hazy, and what I remember are clinical situations, not people. In ordinary surgery certain patients simply faded from one's awareness: these were the patients who only had their dying ahead of them. They were no longer your business. In my nine years of surgery I never heard any discussion about the care of the dying, the emphasis was on maximizing efficiency, technical innovation and high patient turnover.

Whether or not doctors recognize that death occurs, patients continue to die in hospital (or in other institutions if the junior doctor is energetic enough) or else at home. It makes me uncomfortable to think of all those patients in wards where I have worked who must have known in them-selves that they were dying but that I, in my ignorance and immaturity, would not let them speak to me. It must be a terrible agony to know that you are dying and to be surrounded by people (hospital staff and family) who will not allow you to speak about it. It is these deaths that I call 'bad' deaths.

By contrast, the 'good' deaths are memorable for the people rather than for the clinical circumstances of their ends. Those who will allow themselves to do so can learn so much from the dying, and I feel the quality of my experience of living has been enriched by close contacts I have had with people during their time of dying. On the other hand such contact can be profoundly disturbing if the dying person is aggressively denying the reality of his own impending death, or else is being deprived of the opportunity to work through the experience openly.

An experience of someone's dying which moved me and taught me a great deal came during the last months of a psychotherapist with whom I did some of my training. She was in her mid-seventies when an inoperable intestinal cancer was discovered by chance, but she was to live for another 18 months. When talking of her illness she could be distressed like anyone else about the appearance of skin nodules or a pleural effusion. At another level she struggled hard to comprehend the meaning of the cancer inside her. 'Since it is part of me', she would say, 'I cannot treat it as an enemy. Yet it cannot be called a friend. I find it very puzzling'. She never to my knowledge came to a satisfying understanding of the meaning of the cancer but that was really a secondary issue to her concern with the great mystery of death itself.

In an interview some nine months before she died she revealed where she was in her search for understanding.

> I feel in the hands of the living God . . . I don't know why this thing — I suppose it's an evil thing — has taken hold of my body . . . I puzzle about it, and I feel very lonely when I'm with it in isolation, as though it was some 'thing' that was here. But I'm amazed that in a sense it hasn't touched my spirit. I don't understand this. I feel emotionally disturbed from time to time when I just don't feel at all well, and perhaps I have done a little too much and I feel very poorly, and can hardly get myself into bed or up in the morning. And then I can weep to myself — very seldom to others — but I feel my destiny goes on.
>
> I have no less sense of the value of eternity in time because I have a fatal disease, because a lot of the dying I have done already. And a lot of the experience of the eternal has happened to me already, so that in a sense I feel life now . . . In the eternity of now . . . Eternity is here.

She continued to practice until about two weeks before she died. Then she became rapidly weaker, but she was ready to go. On my last visit to her in her old stone cottage in the Cotswolds, she lay in bed and gestured to the garden where the fruit trees were in blossom and the birds were singing.

She said: It's all the same. It all goes on' She repeated this several times as though she had already started on her journey. She was calm yet remote, and when the time came for her to want to be alone once more, she held out her hand for me to kiss because she did not now want anyone closer to her than that.

Ten or twenty years ago a fatal illness in a friend would probably have caused me to retreat from that person. In hospital the care of the dying was simply never discussed so there was no opportunity to develop proper attitudes in the course of my work, and my personal life did not happen to provide opportunities either. When I look back and try to identify at what point in time my attitudes changed, I suspect that until quite recently I probably avoided contact with the dying wherever possible. Of course I could face dying people, that is an inevitable part of any doctor's work, but there is a difference between being able to talk with someone about his impending death and being able to be truly with that person and to share the experience as far as any outsider can. Elisabeth Kübler-Ross catches the quality of this sharing in the closing passages of her book *On Death and Dying*:[15]

> There is a time in a patient's life when the mind slips off into a dreamless state, when the need for food becomes minimal and the awareness of the environment all but disappears into darkness ... Those who have the strength and the love to sit with a dying patient in the *silence that goes beyond words* will know that this moment is neither frightening nor painful, but a peaceful cessation of the functioning of the body. Watching a peaceful death of a human being reminds us of a falling star; one of a million lights in a vast sky that flares up for a brief moment only to disappear into the endless night forever. To be a therapist to a dying patient makes us aware of the uniqueness of each individual in this vast sea of humanity. It makes us aware of our finiteness, our limited lifespan. Few of us live beyond our three score and ten years and yet in that brief time most of us create and live a unique biography and weave ourselves into the fabric of human history.

When I hear doctors offer the hollow generalization that the great majority of people do not want to know when they have a fatal illness, I feel they are merely describing their own difficulties in facing the reality of death. When they say that patients do not ask the fateful question they are quite right, but they do not realize that their attitude communicates to the patient the message that such questions would not be in order. Unfortunately, some medical teams collectively manage to deny death so effectively that they would almost have one believe that whatever else happened in their units patients certainly did not die there. Sometimes the topic: 'What should patients be told about their illnesses?' is discussed. Even that question avoids the central issue. What should really be discussed is: 'How much truth can the doctor stand?'

The process of dying is different from the agony of the first realization of incurable illness, yet the dying is what it is all about. Anyone who has had the privilege of being close to someone who has died in the peace of his own home after a life in which most of the major ambitions have been realized and the personal relationships have been calmly resolved will find the anonymous furtive, technologically dominated hospital death an affront to human dignity.

By what right do doctors and nurses control the manner of dying for the half or even two-thirds of the population of England and Wales which now dies in hospital? It is one of the most bizarre aspects of medical power, and it is an indication of the intensity of the doctors' anxiety concerning death that such preposterous practices continue.

Among the younger doctors, who anyway come from a generation which is more in contact with its feelings, there is a deep sense of dismay at what they see going on in hospitals but in their junior roles they often feel powerless to do anything. But they can sit with the dying in the 'silence that goes beyond words'. They can allow themselves to feel their anxieties about their own mortality, and learn to stay in the uncomfortableness that such awareness brings. They can also learn to tune in to their rationalizations to avoid facing the person who is dying: pressure of other business, fatigue from having been up most of the previous night, adjustment of the dying person's intravenous regimen. Then they can talk to the dying person about dying, after all it is the matter which dominates his thinking. Some dying people can give

sustenance to the living; some need to keep such energies as
they have within themselves. For a dying person the whole of
existence is now. The past is gone and cannot be altered, and
striving can no longer achieve anything. The future is
unknowable, so the reality is in the present moment, and the
doctor may have to make great efforts to shed his Western
progress-orientated attitudes to concentrate his being in the
Now.

In general a psychotherapist can help people according to
the extent of his own development. The dying person has an
experience which I have not had so I am humbled in his
presence. I can share this feeling of humility with him but I
believe that I can still help so long as my feelings are right.
Reading about the business of dying can be a help. Elisabeth
Kübler-Ross[15] describes five stages through which most
people can pass as they come to terms with the actuality of
their death: denial and isolation, anger, bargaining,
depression, acceptance. Some never get beyond the first
stage. People can be helped along towards calm acceptance
but no one can be forced to go further than is right for him.
She illuminates her theme with extended transcripts of interviews with dying patients which can be reassuring to anyone
wanting to work with the dying but not knowing quite how
to begin.

JoAnn Kelley Smith[17] has described her own dying. She
was in her late forties when she developed extensive
secondary deposits from cancer of the breast. She was the
mother of three children, foster mother to several more, and
they all lived together in a small community. She called her
book *Free Fall* because

> the parachute jump comes closest to describing where I am. It is an
> ecstatic falling because you are in space — free of time and all
> restraints. As long as I have little or no pain, my dying is a freeing
> experience . . . But at the same time I'm all alone and the farther I
> fall, the more lonely I feel.

Speaking to her community, she pleaded:

> Don't separate yourselves from me no matter how ugly I become
> either in disposition or in appearance. Don't fail to see me because
> you won't know what to say or because you might cry, or for any
> other excuse you might discover to escape my presence . . . From

this point on I really need you because I feel suspended in space — so lonely that it almost overwhelms me.

When I die, my husband loses his wife, his lover, his confidante. My children lose their mother. Each friend loses me as a friend. But I lose all human relationships. That's the meaning of the free fall. That's the meaning of being alone.

Not only does my free fall separate me from others, but there is a sense in which I am also separated from the person I used to be. To a certain extent I am dead already, for about all I have left are limited creativity and relationships ... As I become more limited, then more of me dies.

For me, death is not just the end of breathing or the moment my heart stops beating, but a process. While there is a sense in which all of our bodies are in this process, for me death began in December of 1972 when I was consciously aware that no only was my body disintegrating, but also my person. I can no longer function as I did. It's not there any more. Those ways are gone. That's death.

JoAnn Smith had prepared herself for death but she did not die as expected for she had a remission of her disease perhaps as a result of intensive chemotherapy which made her hair fall out. She lingered on for months during which she had time to observe her negative emotions as well: her irritability, her tendency to manipulate others or to play on feelings that 'you'll be sorry about that when I'm gone', her 'uncooperativeness' occasionally with her medical advisers. She describes her feelings in great detail yet with directness and simplicity. The reader shares her steady decline with her, and the reader will never again pass by a dying patient in a hospital bed. She also has words for those who want to help.[18]

To have someone cry with me is the most affirming experience I know. It says, 'I know you must feel bad — and because I care about you, I feel bad too'. And if a person stays with me, eventually he will find the clue that can help him deal with some of the deepest needs I am only going to express to another human who can show me that he, too, feels. I know I can trust that person. And he will be able to help ...

When anyone comes to visit me, I don't want him to come with his own agenda ... I often get the feeling that before people enter my room, they try to decide what to say. I don't want to hear their concerns. I want them to empty their heads of their own ideas. When you visit a sick person, fill your head with thoughts about that person, your care for him, and what you can do to get in touch with him.

Sick people, especially most dying people, are very unpleasant to be around and so we avoid visiting them. I know because I was one who always avoided seeing them if I possibly could. I always rationalised to myself, 'Well, I wouldn't know what to say'. But you don't need to say anything. If you just go in and listen, they'll do all the 'saying' because they really want to talk about themselves. And they need to talk about themselves. They need to get in touch with their feelings and they need to tell it to another human.

Looking after a dying person involves caring. Knowledge, skill, experience will not help much. There is little opportunity to impress colleagues and juniors. Relatives in all probability will take what is done for granted. The dying person will be at peace so if the caring doctor has been able to contribute anything it will be in helping to achieve calm — absence of distress. Busy staff may not even notice, in the way they would notice a dramatic cure. Doctors do not describe their dying patients at clinical meetings. The rewards are private.

Looking after or being with a dying person may be called an example of simple caring. I believe that the doctor who can care for the dying is potentially the best doctor, not only because he can give of himself but also because he transcends the curing role.

Those who have in any way come close to death thereafter speak in a special way about life, and manage to live fully in the Eternal Everchanging Present, taking each day as it comes. I would find it hard to savour the richness of summer without reference to the winter that preceded it and which will follow it. Day would be hard to imagine without night. As I become more aware of death because I am getting older and encounter more people who are dying, so life becomes richer. This is not because each day I move nearer to the end of my life but rather because the reality of death intensifies the reality of living.

Summary

Problems which arise in connection with the care of the dying have been examined in the light of the doctor's personal attitudes to death. This is highlighted by the divergence of views between doctors and patients about how much people should know about their fatal illnesses. The unhappy situation is unlikely to change until doctors can face their own anxieties concerning their own mortality. The doctor who can sustain a dying person is potentially the best doctor.

DOCTORS

11. The Honoured Practitioner

The emerging doctor

In 1966, 76% of entrants to medical school in Britain came from the professional and managerial classes (social classes 1 and 2), but only 18% of the working population belonged to those classes. At the other end of the scale only 2.5% of entrants came from the lower two social classes (4 and 5) which comprised 32% of the working population.[1]

In those days medical students seemed a curiously, almost anachronistically, conservative and conforming group. There were no sartorial constraints on the clinical students, but they were generally more neatly turned out, and with shorter hair, than most of their contemporaries. They were deferential, addressed their teachers as 'Sir', and seldom expressed any fundamental criticisms of society or the medical profession. They gave a general impression that they enjoyed the prospect of becoming part of a great profession.

There seemed to be certain similarities between many of the attitudes of these students and those of what has been called the 'authoritarian personality',[2] a concept which emerged out of an inquiry into the roots of anti-semitism, and refers to a wide-ranging attitude of intolerance and illiberality. The authoritarian tends to identify with the existing social order and establishment organizations (including the church) and so resists change or any outsiders or minority groups which might be imagined to threaten it. He adopts a tough-minded approach to human problems.

dislikes expressions of emotion and introspection but may reveal a streak of superstition. He will probably favour corporal and capital punishment and will be especially severe towards any sexual indulgence or drug abuse. Most importantly, he accepts the dictates of authority, whether they come from parents, teachers or political leaders (from the right or the left as the case may be), and will change — even totally reverse — his stoutly held beliefs when told to do so by a suitable authority figure.

These underlying attitudes suspected in many of the students seem to me at the present time to be manifest in the medical profession when viewed collectively. Furthermore, many of the complaints about the arrogance and unapproachability of doctors seem comprehensible in these terms. The authoritarian profile (and it is intended as a profile, not as a precise description) fits the collective image of all the established professions, but it fits doctors peculiarly well. If these authoritarian tendencies which seem to be present in qualified doctors were also present in medical students it would suggest that the profession was attracting those who identified with the traditional (authoritarian) image of the doctor, and so would tend to perpetuate them when qualified.

Authoritarian attitudes can be identified by fairly straightforward questions, and so a colleague and I in the late 1960s drew up an *ad hoc* questionnaire along these lines which we gave to first year students in psychology, philosophy, languages, history, mechanical engineering and, of course, medicine. It was no more than a pilot enquiry and is not offered as evidence but the authoritarian tendencies were much more pronounced among the medicals than among those in the arts faculty, with the mechanical engineers in between but veering towards the medicals' attitudes.

The underlying dispositions of young people have been intensively studied by an imaginative psychologist, Liam Hudson, who has identified what he has called 'convergers' and 'divergers'.[3] Convergers are, broadly speaking, those who do better at straightforward intelligence tests as compared with open-ended tests where there is no single correct answer. They prefer exactness, are intolerant of ambiguity and tend to avoid expressions of emotion and opportunities to use their imaginative powers. They are not only ready to accept authority, but they will seek out those courses of study where the body of factual information and the weight of accepted authority is greatest. The diverger is the opposite in almost all these respects, and in the educational system is more likely to be found studying the humanities. Hudson[4] has also shown that the convergers tends to display the authoritarian tendencies particularly with regard to the acceptance of the teaching and attitudes of their elders.

These convergent tendencies can appear as early as 15 or 16 years[4] before any clear choice of career is made. The schoolboy (most of Hudson's work seems to have been done on boys) then selects a course of study which conforms with his disposition, and selects an occupation which has a public image that similarly matches his convergent temperament. The emergence of the diverger is less precise and his tendencies do not manifest themselves as definitely or as early on.

Hudson does not deal specifically with medical students but I feel his work is completely applicable to them. It would suggest that the student comes to medical school with a set of very definite ideas about the content and structure of the medical course, and about the kind of person he aims to become once he is qualified. This certainly was the gloomy reality as I experienced it from medical students in the late 1960s, as did others engaged in trying to introduce something of the social sciences into the medical curriculum.[5,6] 'We came here to study scientific medicine, and you are trying to teach us about human relationships. What have they got to do with science?' This quite common utterance was sometimes a taunt, but sometimes a question arising out of a quite genuine bewilderment at the ambiguities inherent in any study of human relationships.

This was all a fair time ago. There is still a bias towards sons and daughters of professional people, and the academic requirements for entry have been stiffened up out of all recognition, but there has been a profound change in attitudes: there is now a much greater social awareness amongst pre-clinical students, and groups of these students

have taken on part-time hospital and social work in a way
which would have been unheard of ten years ago. The
vociferous conservatives are still there but they have been
joined by the vociferous radicals. When they get to the wards,
however, the latter quickly learn when to conceal this social
awareness, if only because in many cases the good jobs are in
the gift of those who do not welcome this broader approach.
The young doctor may be in something of a dilemma in that
his liberal attitudes may well impede his progress towards the
secure, high status life which is now a visible reality to him.
(It is not unique to medicine that the radical student
becomes conformist once it seems that he may suffer
materially on account of his protest.)

The virtuoso role

Most people have indulged in the fantasy of being the possessor of a dazzling talent which can enthrall thousands, or the
hero who intervenes dramatically and saves the situation. For
the vast majority this can only ever be a fantasy: for the
doctor, if he so chooses, it can be a daily reality. It is a
beguiling possibility to be able to become a hero at will and
with no danger to oneself, and it is very good for the development of a clear sense of identity and personal worth. It is
so tempting in fact that few doctors can resist it, for a short
period of their career at any rate.

The opportunity to enjoy the virtuoso role has become
possible because of the colossal success of medicine since the
middle of the nineteenth century. Before that time the
physician had a lower status in the social hierarchy, and the
surgeon (who did the messy manual work) and the apothe-
cary (who handled the medicines) were even further down
the scale. Nowadays, with the pre-eminence of technology,
technical knowledge and manual dexterity have overtaken
human qualities as gatherers of prestige, and so the surgeon
has now been elevated to the position of highest regard.

Some of the qualities which go to make up the professional virtuoso have been brought together by the sociologist
Peter Nokes[7] and they will be set out, slightly modified,
below.

Social distance

The operatic prima donna requires an orchestra and supporting cast, the ship's captain requires a crew, the surgeon requires operating theatre assistants. These distinctive performers are nothing without their background personnel, indeed they only achieve their full identity against this background, but almost as important as their background is their distance from it. The virtuoso has to stand alone.

In medicine, surgical virtuosity attained its zenith in the early years of this century when the surgeon was often the only really skilled person present in the operating theatre. Nowadays, the social distance implied in that situation has weakened because of the presence of anaesthetists, technicians and other highly competent persons, but it has by no means disappeared whatever *bonhomie* the casual visitor might observe.

Special skills

Doctors can respond serenely to the most vigorous criticisms of their profession because they know that this criticism will cease abruptly the moment someone falls ill, or even fears the possibility of illness. The fact that the techniques called for on such occasions may be simple in no way weakens the authority of their possessor. Indeed most of the skills commonly used are elementary, so much so that it is widely suggested that much of the general practitioner's work could be done by people without a full medical qualification. In less developed countries this is certainly true, but a large proportion of the overworked doctors in this country stoutly resist any suggestions along these lines, and terms like 'barefoot doctor' and *'feldscher'* are treated with suspicion. In psychiatric work an even greater proportion of the routine work can be done as well, and in many cases better, by non-medically qualified workers, but they too are treated with suspicion accompanied with murmurings about confidentiality, 'clinical responsibility' and the dangers of unrecognized brain tumours.

Doctors want the work-loads reduced but they are not

prepared to risk their virtuoso status as the possessors of special skills. I think they are mistaken in this fear. No matter how much of the regular work is done by others, they have so much more basic and theoretical knowledge covering such a wide area, and the all-important ability to cope with the major crisis, that there will always be a contribution for the medically trained to make.

Esoteric knowledge

The public's desire for information makes many doctors acutely uncomfortable, and they can describe technical details to a patient so badly that they give the impression they do not understand what they are talking about. The patient then misunderstands what has been said, thereby confirming the doctor's view that patients cannot understand explanations. Doctors do not always want to share information, hence the offensive slogan still emblazoned on some British hospital case note folders: 'Not to be Handled by the Patient'. The most junior member of staff may peruse this document which may contain the patient's death sentence, often in the presence of the patient, but the patient is not allowed to see it.

Until medical sociologists and writers like Paul Ferris[8] came along, the medical profession had maintained the illusion that not only could non-medically qualified people never comprehend medical matters but they could not even comprehend the administration of medical care: only doctors can understand doctoring was the theme. The new breed of non-medical hospital administrators have shown painfully well that they can understand the minutiae of medical care, and with a clarity that is not quite appreciated by the old guard of doctors.

However, as with the question of special skills, there is little for the doctors to worry about. Medical technology is advancing so fast and in so many different directions that few non-medical technologists could grasp the significance of developments as well as an averagely well-informed doctor. I suspect that the threat implied by working with a medically well-informed public and lay administration is a symbolic threat to the doctor's virtuoso status because of the mistaken belief that he is being deprived of his store of esoteric knowledge.

Manifest disaster factor

Many kinds of experts can intervene dramatically: few but doctors can intervene dramatically and demonstrate by their critical act that their initiative alone made all the difference. Surgeons do it all the time, and so all the time their special status is being reinforced. Furthermore, the more dramatic the intervention the more dramatic is the background of possible disaster. The surgeon always works with the possibility that one false move can lead to catastrophe.

The true virtuoso has to generate the feeling in those around him that his intervention — on his terms and on nobody else's — is vital to the health and the very survival of the patient. Doctors collectively use these strategies to ensure that their recommendations alone are followed in the planning of health care, but non-medical administrators call this 'shroud waving', and pay less attention to it than they used to.

Medical temples

Medicine is so complex and requires such advanced equipment that it can only really be practised in special places. This is an inevitable consequence of advanced technological medicine because all the machinery has to be housed and maintained somewhere. Any threat to the traditional role of the doctor is more than compensated for by these temples so long as advanced technology is assumed to be good and to be in the patient's best interest.

The virtuoso role is naturally an agreeable one, particularly for the doctor who enjoys it simply by belonging to a particular profession, and does not have to keep on scoring triumphs in order to perpetuate it. All that is required is that some members of the profession do keep on scoring goals, but the media can be relied upon to make the most of every 'breakthrough' and 'wonder drug' because of the public's insatiable appetite for such details. The public wants heroes, so I doubt if doctors are really more than rather pleasantly meeting a widely felt need.

Is the virtuoso role necessary for the proper discharge of the doctor's clinical function? Is it even desirable? Some doctors feel that it is essential for the clinician to establish himself as a figure on whom the ailing patient can rely, someone who is totally confident and in command of the situation. This is attractive to the inexperienced as they can envelop themselves in an armour of impenetrable calm, and so provide support in all circumstances.

Teamwork, among a variety of professionals, in the community as well as in hospital, is gradually replacing the solo medical practitioner, and there will be a weakening of the obvious virtuoso role. It remains to be seen how the medical profession adapts to this change. In the future doctors may try to practise a more open, less charismatic kind of medicine in partnership with a well-informed public, or they may develop new strategies so as to keep their talents permanently on display.

Power and prestige

Doctors are permitted by society to do things to people, even with a knife provided it is called a scalpel, which would otherwise be punished by imprisonment or even death. When patients die on the operating table searching questions are seldom asked, and until experimental surgeons overstepped the mark with certain transplant operations it seemed that the more advanced and hazardous the procedure the better the public liked it. I never attracted such instant awe and respect at cocktail parties as when I was working at cardio-thoracic surgery with its horrifying mortality, whereas few people were much interested in my activities of the year before when I was providing basic surgical care for an under-nourished population in Libya.

There is a unique authority contained in the right to kill people, and it is backed up by a number of lesser powers sanctioned by the state by virtue of having a medical qualification. This is a right doctors possess for as long as they live, without any need for periodic review unless they draw attention to themselves by gross professional incompetence.

The great majority of doctors are not consciously seeking power; on the other hand almost everyone enjoys respect and prestige. The power vested in doctors determines the way they are regarded by society, and they reap great benefits from society. Doctors expect to be treated as something special. They expect to be able to park their cars where they will, or to have a telephone installed promptly, or to receive special attention in shops because of an unspoken but implicit sense of clinical urgency which the public want to believe and which doctors do not care to disown.

The authority of the doctor is a complex matter, and cannot be formulated in terms of power alone, but whatever the origins of our authority it is manifestly there. Because doctors all benefit from it they cannot claim to be uninvolved, and they should assume that they have an interest in perpetuating this power.

Withholding information

> A physician's ability to preserve his own power over the patient in the doctor-patient relationship depends largely on his ability to control the patient's uncertainty. The physician enhances his power to the extent that he can maintain the patient's uncertainty about the course of illness, efficacy of therapy, or specific future actions of the physician himself.[9]

This is a proposition devised by two Harvard workers from the sociological idea that: 'the power of A over B depends on A's ability to predict B's behavior and on the uncertainty of B about A's behavior'.

It is not being suggested that patients are deliberately kept in a state of ignorance but simply that the doctor's life is easier if the patient remains uninformed. There is a paradox between the doctor confidently and gravely advising his patient to accept his treatment, and the same doctor embroiled in an academic free-for-all with his colleagues about the merits and demerits of this self-same treatment. If doctors explained everything to every patient it would soon become apparent how often doctors simply do not know; thus witholding information has the double advantage of keeping the patient pliable through the anxiety of uncertainty, and keeping the myth of medical omniscience intact through never revealing ignorance.

Encouraging passivity and regression

The cheerful, calm, willing, and appreciative patient is even easier to control than the ignorant one and he also feeds the doctor's appetite for appreciation. Everybody tends to regress when ill; indeed, it is a tendency we all have at times of crisis but when it has been decided that we are ill it becomes socially acceptable.

Everyone wants to believe that his doctor is not only competent but extra-specially good, or maybe the cleverest doctor in the locality. In other words he wants to believe that his doctor possesses great powers because it is comforting to feel that one is in the best hands. People respect power in others, and all the more so when it is working for one's personal benefit. Thus the doctor's already real power may be augmented if the patient invests him with yet more attributes of potency and skill, and then intensifies the process further by slipping into a state of helpless passivity. This kind of regressive behaviour may be permissible in brief minor illnesses but it is the very antithesis of what is required in highly technological medical procedures such as haemodialysis[10] when an active informed participation is vital.

Dangers of power and prestige

Power for the doctor means that he has the unchallenged right to work as he likes. The greatest single danger of this is that his personal peculiarities, prejudices and blind spots will proliferate unchecked. Anyone under any psychological pressure or anyone who finds himself in a situation which

touches his sensitive areas — whether or not these are consciously recognized — is liable to react by avoiding having to
face these painful matters squarely. If that person is all-
powerful then no-one can point out his foibles to him. The
Shakespearean type of court jester, who alone can ridicule
the king, has no modern counterpart, although I believe the
Pope still has a confessor who is a simple priest. Doctors may
work in groups but these are nearly always implicitly competitive associations whether for resources or simply for
professional prestige. Michael Balint[11] started his general
practitioner groups partly to meet problems like these. They
made a great impact on medical thinking but no so much on
practice, because the doctors who would derive the greatest
benefit from such an opportunity to reveal themselves do not
go to groups, nor do they recognize that such outlets could
be of any value to them.

One of the dangers is that the doctor comes to believe that
he possesses great wisdom and competence. He works
tremendously long hours because he thinks that the service
could not run properly without him, and that he is in
enormous personal demand. Patients must not therefore be
surprised if they are kept waiting for long periods, and if he
is a hospital doctor he will have generated a lengthy waiting
list to consolidate his view of himself. His feelings of self-
importance can delude him into thinking that he has special
insights and therefore can express dogmatic opinions about
everything, including personal morality. He may also come
to *live through his patients.* He has probably managed to
establish a style of working where his patients have to accept
him uncritically, and finds that their company makes few
emotional demands on him. Eventually he cannot tolerate
anyone close to him who is not dependent. Family life
suffers and the doctor experiences life vicariously through his
patients, enjoying their successes, their love affairs and even
their failures. Indeed such a doctor is in danger of holding on
to patients through his need to live his life through them.[12]

These types of behaviour are really quite common among
all kinds of doctors, and they seem to be manifestations of a
sense of power. There is a great need of patients but the need
can evolve into a need to dominate. Thus such a doctor is

not likely to make the kind of relationship in which a patient will be facilitated in developing any potential he may have for helping himself. The very opposite in fact because this kind of doctor will only tolerate passive compliance.

Why any doctor should evolve in this direction in the first place cannot be explained with any certainty. I suspect, however, that many of the undesirable developments in a doctor's style of living and working, particularly where power is concerned, arise from difficulties the doctor has had in the direct relationship with patients. The close involvement in other people's lives was not something that a medical training in the past had led young doctors to expect to meet, let alone to have to cope with. These doctors with authoritarian attitudes and little capacity for making empathic relationships of a non-sexual kind found themselves in intimate confrontation with patients in distress. Their medical knowledge was of no help to them because ultimately distressed people or those desperately worried about the implications of an illness want not information but human support, and that kind of simple direct expression of caring is something I fear doctors were, and to a great extent still are, curiously inept at giving. One reason for this may be that they belong to that school of thought (or school of defence) in medicine which demands that the doctor must at all times be above the vicissitudes of human experience, and so in practice the patient must forever be held off at a distance.

Professional dangers. It is sad that relatively few doctors, or other professionals, manage to derive lasting satisfaction from the actual work they were trained to do. So many branch out into sidelines which in the end consume more of their mental and emotional energy than their main professional work. Doctors have such autonomy in their work (however much they complain about administrative interference), that if their main activity becomes unsatisfying, and they cannot find a new and positive attitude towards it, they can always branch out into other fields. Unfortunately, the fields usually chosen lead them away from the principal task and into the deserts of medical politics and administration. Membership of committees is then sought as the ladder to office and public distinction in the many medical organizations which flourish wherever doctors are gathered together in any numbers.

In Britain there is the British Medical Association, the Society of Apothecaries, The Royal Colleges of Physicians—Surgeons—Obstetricians and Gynaecologists—Pathologists—Psychiatrists—Radiologists, etc., but these organizations have made little contribution to medicine as the business of caring for sick people. They have provided an absorbing and clinically wasteful outlet for large numbers of doctors who cannot resist the ceremonial trappings, which then become confused in their own minds with professional competence and authority.

We then have the pathetic and dangerous spectacle of 'the honoured scientist'. This is Solzhenitzyn's term for the academic doctor and all who seek institutional distinction in professional organizations.

> ... if a man was called a Scientist during his lifetime and an Honoured one at that, it was the end of him as a doctor. The honour and glory of it would get in the way of his treatment of his patients, just as elaborate clothing hinders a man's movements. These Honoured Scientists went about with a suite of followers, like some new Christ with his apostles. They completely lost the right to make mistakes or not to know something, they lost the right to be allowed to think things over. The man might be self-satisfied, half-witted, behind the times, and trying to conceal the fact, and yet everyone would expect miracles from him.

Solzhenitsyn[13] was writing out of his own experiences in hospital in Tashkent in Central Asia. He could as well have been writing about every doctor's own teaching hospital.

Summary

The person of the doctor is of fundamental importance in the delivery of health care. Medical students display 'authoritarian' tendencies during their school years which may lead them into medicine in the first place, and which may cause them to perpetuate the autocratic image of the medical profession.

The concept of the virtuoso is applied to the doctor as a way of establishing a position of power and prestige in society. Then some of the ways this power may be perpetuated are described, such as by withholding information and encouraging passivity and regression, and also some of the dangers of these habits for the doctor at a personal level as well as in his professional life.

12. Doctors in Private

The urbane practitioner who can cope with every clinical crisis, who can comfort the frightened and distressed, calm and help resolve the most painful domestic conflicts, and who can sustain the hopeless and the bereaved, has another life in which the same dramas are enacted. In this life he is no longer the outside benefactor but an active participant.

There is no reason to suppose that his skills in his professional life will help him to deal with the same problems among his family and friends. Indeed the reverse may be the case, so that the more experienced he is, the higher his status, and the more he is admired by his patients the greater may be the gulf between his professional and his domestic life, between his professional self and his private self.

Professional mask

The average doctor has to play so many different roles that it is hard to find out which one represents the 'real' person, if indeed the idea of there being a real person, or real self, has any true meaning. On the surface, however, there is undoubtedly a professional self, which almost everyone finds necessary for a number of good reasons.

Personal identity

Personal identity is the individual's perception of who he is

147

and what he can do. Medical students, like all others around the age of 18, are actively though unconsciously engaged in forming their personal identity. This is a necessary process because if it is not accomplished the adolescent will never become emancipated from parents to become an independent member of society and a confident member of one or other sex.

The medical student, unlike students of the humanities, acquires an identity along with his education by his identification with the medical profession. He may be a rebellious student but he will be working in a large building called the Medical School and an even larger one called the Teaching Hospital, which by their very bulk and implied power impose themselves on the uncertain, emerging adult. The mystique of belonging to a great profession, epitomised in some of the writings of William Osler[1] — who was the apotheosis of the erudite, paternalistic physician — is currently out of favour, but membership of the medical profession can still be very convenient on occasions, especially when times are hard or when one is in some difficulty or other far from home.

Coping with the world, and personal protection

Part of growing up in any society involves 'socializing' which means conforming and delaying gratification. It also involves developing some armour to protect our private selves from the batterings of other people, so that we can proceed on our way through life without daily being wounded intentionally or accidentally. Even at school the medical student may have had to suppress his feelings during classes for animal dissection, and later too when confronted with the for-malinized bodies in the anatomy department. But the greatest need for protection comes when first encountering the sufferings and tragedies which are part of the routine on any hospital ward.

So often the medical students, and junior doctors too, react with a robust kind of detachment, so that grave or gruesome matters are the subject of jokes. A student working

on a radiotherapy ward was once able to tell me trium-
phantly: 'it's great on this ward, because we don't have to
get up at night to resuscitate them if they arrest!' One of the
consequences of behavioural science teaching, and of
students and junior doctors becoming more aware of psychosocial factors, is that the human realities of illness can no
longer be totally disregarded. Doctors are being made more
aware of these psychosocial factors but they are not as yet
being given the support they need to carry some of the
emotional burdens that have thereby been generated for
them.

To refer to patients as 'the abscess' or 'the stomach' or,
even worse, to clinically uninteresting patients as 'rubbish',
may only reflect the doctor's need for protection.

Doctors' afflictions

The public like to tell doctors that they have high rates for
illness — especially myocardial infarction — and the
possibility of an early death from suicide or the consequences
of heavy drinking. The implication of these claims (or taunts)
is that doctors work under greater pressure and for longer
hours than other groups in the community, and that they
become overwhelmed by the daily company they keep with
misery and suffering. Doctors cannot fail to be interested in
matters relating to their own health but recognize that
blanket statistical statements applied to large numbers of
diverse characters are not likely to describe one's special case.
However, there are several questions which are worth
examining.

Psychological problems of doctors

Personal distress is such a private matter that to try to
quantify it in order to make some general statements is
likely to produce irrelevancies. However, there are some
useful indicators of a person's state of well being, such as
manifest psychological symptoms, severe marital problems
and divorce, regular consultations with a psychiatrist,
alcoholism and drug abuse and suicide.

These have all been the subject of considerable study and the general conclusion is that doctors make a pretty poor showing. The studies are mainly statistical and therefore they disagree over details but the overall trends stand out clearly. What seems to me to be important is not exactly where doctors stand on the ladder of psychosocial distress in contemporary society, but the fact that they lead lives no better integrated than those of the people they are employed to treat and sustain. This paradox as much as anything else justifies the special scrutiny being given to doctors in these four chapters.

Manifest psychological disorder. The impaired judgement of a doctor over a period of several months can cause an immense amount of avoidable distress, and avoidable deaths as well. Unfortunately the professional competence of doctors has hardly been studied at all although their breakdowns have been extensively documented.

It is salutary therefore to have the experiences of three New York and New Jersey psychiatrists[2] concerning 13 doctors under their care who at times had been less than a credit to their profession. Here are some extracts from their account.

> A surgeon . . . rewrote house-staff orders because he believed that the orders had been written to embarrass him.

> A physician tormented his patients with unnecessary diagnostic tests, always doubting that he had done enough. As a house officer, he had spent hours attempting to revive deceased patients.

Another physician was proved to have

> consistently falsified medical data. For example, when instructed to watch a bleeding patient throughout the night, he did not do so, entering bogus hematocrit data in the chart at a convenient time the next day. He never showed any remorse when confronted with evidence of fraudulent activity.

> A profoundly depressed internist flattered his patients by confiding in them, but some admitted that they could not tell him about their troubles since *his* troubles occupied so much of the consulting time.

A young physician's comments at meetings

were often incomprehensible to others, but they assumed that they simply failed to grasp his humour or imagination, and that he practiced good medicine, since he was well read and well informed. His strange comments were an illustration of a schizophrenic thought disorder, reflecting unusual associations, autism, and idiosyncratic thinking.

A physician who appeared to have had a successful result from cancer surgery dealt with fears of recurrence by the defence of denial . . . He minimised his patients' complaints and failed to investigate potentially dangerous symptoms.

A surgeon said that he believed in telling the truth to his patients. He gratified his sadistic impulses by emphasising the least likely and gravest possible outcome of patients' illnesses.

Most authors who have investigated the problem of mentally sick doctors have tended to bracket together conventional psychiatric symptomatology, alcoholism and drug addition.[3-10] Their samples are inevitably special and their diagnostic criteria vary, but certain themes stand out. In a substantial proportion there was evidence of psychological difficulties during the student years. The most likely time for actual breakdown seems to be in the doctor's late thirties, when he is really becoming established professionally, but there is usually a history of several years of personal distress before the actual break. No medical specialty was consistently over-represented.

Doctors seem slow to recognize when a colleague is floundering on account of his psychological difficulties, at least they are slow to acknowledge this fact clearly and openly, and to stop covering up for his shortcomings. It is a variation of the tendency to avoid diagnosing malignant disease in a colleague. However, once the problem has been recognized, doctors get good support, although they can make difficult patients, with a high proportion terminating their treatment against advice. Some reports complain at the doctor-patients wanting to 'interfere' with treatment programmes, but some[8] see this as a positive aspect. A good proportion get back to professional work but often there is a reorientation away from the more hectic kinds of practice, and it seems that the recovering doctors often receive great help from their colleagues in the process of reintegration.

One study by George Vaillant and his colleagues[9] from Cambridge, Massachusetts, is of especial interest because it reflects the general findings, and because its subjects and controls were followed up for 30 years. It began as an investigation of 268 male students who were selected on the grounds of good health and satisfactory academic progress. Details of early life were obtained by means of a home visit, and the subjects were contacted thereafter at two-yearly intervals. 47 of the students attended medical school, and two-thirds of them were at Columbia, Harvard, Johns Hopkins, Pennsylvania and Rochester; all but one graduated. They were compared with a group of 79 'socio-economically matched controls' from the original 268.

Over three-quarters of the doctors had passed their specialty-board examinations, and all were currently 'gainfully employed'. At the time of the investigation when the subjects must have been approaching 50, the authors felt the doctors were probably in better than average general health, yet 47% of the doctors had 'poor marriages' or had been divorced (compared with 32% of the controls); 20% had actually been divorced (controls 14%). 36% reported 'trouble with control' of alcohol, or 'often' used sleeping pills, or had taken amphetamines or tranquillizers daily for more than one month (controls 22%). 34% of the doctors had paid ten or more visits to a psychiatrist (controls 19%).

They found that the subjects and controls who had 'good' backgrounds (warm, supportive homes with good parental relationships) and who were 'psychologically sound' at college had significantly fewer of the problems indicated above. The subjects were divided into two groups according to specialty. Surgeons, administrators and research workers were regarded in this context as not 'having primary responsibility for patient care', and they had symptom patterns and qualities of childhood 'very similar' to those of the controls. The internists, psychiatrists, obstetricians and paediatricians (rather arbitrarily lumped together, the investigators admit) had significantly more 'emotional difficulties during adulthood' and 'instability' during childhood as compared with the other two groups. This trend for the more clinically involved practitioners to have a greater frequency of psychological difficulty crops up in a number of studies perhaps backing up these authors' contention that some doctors 'may elect to assume direct care of patients to give others the care that they did not receive in their own childhoods'. This stands in contrast to the general assumption that the clinically involved doctors have more problems *because* of the physical demands of their work.

Drug addiction. Before the drug explosion of the early 1960s doctors were said to account for about 15% of all addicts, with another 15% contributed by nurses and pharmacists.[11, 12] Many of these addicts functioned at an outwardly satisfactory level and their habit was either unknown to their colleagues or else tacitly accepted. Many of course did not continue to function, but according to one series[11] 7 out of 25 returned to medical practice and claimed to be cured of addiction, which nowadays would be regarded as a high rate of success. Certainly the addicts of those days were a different population from the contemporary drop-out junkie: they tended to be in their late thirties, had married (although there was a high incidence of marital discord, and a tendency for the male addict to be the dependent partner), and had previously coped quite adequately in their medical work. As was common with most addicts of those days, many of the doctor-addicts began the habit after analgesic medication prescribed by another doctor for a painful illness.

With some drugs now more widely available and others much more tightly controlled, the pattern of medical addiction has changed, and it is now so covert that it would be hard to make any generally valid observations: statistics about illegal practices are hardly likely to be accurate. The medical drug user is nowadays in a more precarious position than formerly, and will sometimes try to conceal the habit even though consulting a psychiatrist for personal problems. I had been seeing a doctor on account of a sexual problem for some time when one evening I was telephoned by a Samaritan counsellor from the doctor's flat. I went there to find my colleague in a stuporose condition, and upstairs in the bedroom there were the broken ampoules, a blood-stained syringe and sheets, with a touch of the bizarre in the form of the stethoscope, white coat and medical textbooks. Doctors should benignly be assumed to be as evasive about drug usage as anyone else with the same problem.

The huge turnover, and thus easy availability, of psycho-active drugs in the course of most clinical work nowadays means that doctors must be more careful than ever to avoid self-medication.

Alcoholism.[13] The high mortality rate from cirrhosis of the liver amongst British doctors testifies to the size of the problem in Britain[14,15] and in the United States it is currently estimated that there are around 20 000 alcoholics among the 324 000 doctors there.[16] The heavy drinking doctor is such a familiar figure that nobody bothers much, and his advice will still be sought for minor complaints; doctors and the public are curiously accepting and ready to cover up.

This tendency to cover up must prevent an appreciable number of doctors from receiving help at a stage when they might be expected to benefit from it. Every doctor can look back on his student days, or to his time as a hospital junior, and recollect a few colleagues who were something of a joke because of their liking for alcohol. Twenty or thirty years on they will appear much less than a joke because they may have stumbled into alcoholism with well-meaning colleagues making excuses for them, locums being engaged at short notice when things get too bad, and nothing decisive ever happening to halt the downward slide until there is a scandal — a car crash or a public lapse that cannot be denied. Then, as Griffith Edwards[17] has put it:

> There is an immediate demand that he should be dismissed or retired. His previous work for the hospital is forgotten, and it is discovered that he was never really up to standard. He is referred to a psychiatrist with the expectation that the appropriate report will be furnished which will dispose of him.

It seems to be rare for doctors to get desperately needed help until they draw attention to themselves outside the profession.[16]

The reports dealing with drinking doctors also refer to the

frequency of drug abuse, and so if one of these habits is evident then the other should be suspected also.

Suicide is the ultimate indicator of psychosocial distress. Doctors are assumed to experience more such distress than others, therefore it is expected that they will have the highest rate for suicide. This assumption is supported by quite a large literature[18,19,20] but some of these surveys have been sharply attacked on methodological grounds.[21] It is claimed that the surveys are often based on small samples which are then expressed as death rates per 100 000; and that there is insufficient standardization because doctors anyway fall into a high risk group (predominantly older than average, male, white, living in urban areas, high divorce rates). Of those who seriously intend to kill themselves, doctors (and of course other professionals familiar with the effects of drugs) will be more successful than the average citizen. Thus the suicide figures for the medical profession will be further inflated. A better measure would come from recording the numbers who seriously intended to kill themselves but this information would be impossible to obtain.

Some of the widely quoted studies appear to have been based on little more than newspaper reports, but there are others where good samples have been obtained, for example, 'a computerized review of all death certificates filed in the state of California' for 1959, 1960 and 1961.[20]

In this Californian study the suicide rate for male doctors was more than twice that for similar social class standing, or for the population of the state as a whole. However, doctors still had only the fifth highest rate, being exceeded by 'chemists, dentists, pharmacists, and non-medical technicians'. When 'health-care' workers of all kinds (excluding psychologists) are taken togehter the suicide rate for the men is more than double that of other 'professional–technical' workers, and for the women slightly less than double. As with the population generally, the suicide rate increases with age, but there is a very sudden rise for doctors after the age of 65.

No difference was found between medical specialties although the numbers were small in each group. In other surveys psychiatry has been put at the top of the list[18] but it is far from clear if that is the true picture. If it is, it has then to be asked whether the explanation is to be found in the make-up of those entering psychiatry, the special pressures of that work, or the fact that psychiatrists have the greatest direct experience of the mechanics of suicide and self-injury.

The British government statistics show an unequivocally high rate for doctors as compared with other professionals such as lawyers, school teachers and the clergy, and the population as a whole. The high rate was evident in the ten-year period up to 1961 (before 1961 suicide was a criminal offence in Britain) and ever since.[14,15]

The doctor's special predicament

If, as seems likely, doctors do have high rates for suicide, psychological problems, divorce and marital distress, drug taking and alcoholism, where is any explanation or illumination to be found? The job itself can be scrutinised to see what special pressures prevail upon doctors in the course of their work, and also what opportunities present themselves to render doctors extra vulnerable. Then there is the personality of the doctor himself, and whether or not there are intrinsic factors which make the doctor more liable than others to succumb to any of the predictable pressures of living.

Pressures from medical work. The public like to imagine that doctors work long and irregular hours, with a great deal of dashing about from one urgent case to another, and doctors seldom object to this collective image of themselves. It is of course true that many clinical doctors do lead hectic lives, but so do a great many other people, and so I do not feel a general case can be made that doctors work under a greater stress of time and rapid decision-making than do many other groups. The same goes even for those in competitive private practice where the practitioner has to be readily available at all times.

The particular aspects of medical work which seem to me to distinguish it from nearly all other high pressure professional activities are, first, the continual need to make rapid decisions on which lives may depend, often on the basis of inadequate information. In the course of a busy morning's work numerous decisions are made and action is planned on the basis of probabilities, and only the most likely cause for any symptoms can be considered and followed up. This means that much of the time the doctor is left wondering if he should not have looked more closely for some other possibilities, and I suspect a great deal of anxiety and disillusionment is built up over the years by only being able to deal with the surfaces of things. This is one reason why many doctors like to mix some private practice with their public commitment, so that for some part of their week they can work as slowly and as thoroughly as they feel the circumstances warrant.

Secondly, and more important and specific to medical work, is the daily contact with distress and suffering. The doctor is trained to relieve suffering, and he thinks in terms of removing it rather than helping people to accept it, but of course a great deal of the mental and physical suffering a doctor encounters cannot be relieved. Furthermore, the training most doctors received until very recently (and perhaps their own psychological make-up as well) left them peculiarly ill-prepared to deal with many of the human problems they routinely encounter. They would therefore find themselves confronted not only with suffering they could not relieve but also with manifest personal distress which they had no way of comprehending. It follows as a rider to this that if they cannot recognize personal problems in their patients they are even less likely to recognize them in themselves and in their own domestic circumstances.

Personalities of doctors. From the outside, the medical professional can appear monolithic, with all doctors presenting the same basic image; from within, the profession appears infinitely diverse and it contains a niche for every medically qualified person whatever his disposition. Whatever his habits and tastes, however bizarre his ideal life-style, somewhere in the world he will find his place.

For the breezy extrovert there is orthopaedics and (unfortunately) gynaecology; for the meticulous there is neurosurgery and ophthalmology; for the creative plastic and reconstructive surgery; for the recluse there is the laboratory; for the politically minded any specialty that leaves plenty of time for committees; for the militaristic the armed forces; for the radicals and social misfits psychiatry; for the slightly crazy also psychiatry because working with those more disadvantaged than oneself can be quite therapeutic. All these specialties can be practised in the industrial capitals of the west, and a good many of them in the third world as well. There are ships, from passenger liners to whalers on year-long voyages, and there are always the polar ice-caps.

There is never even any need to go on practising medicine because when a doctor drops out of his profession he becomes extra interesting in his new role: doctor-poet, actor-doctor, entrepreneur-doctor, doctor-priest, doctor-revolutionary, doctor-politician (at the time of writing two African heads-of-state are medically qualified), and even doctor-vagabond.

So diverse are the personalities of established doctors that common factors are only likely to be readily apparent during the student years, certain of which were described in Chapter 11. Nevertheless, studies of mentally ill doctors have repeatedly emphasized the importance of early life experiences in relation to psychosocial difficulties in adult life, and of course in forming the adult personality in the first place.

> Twenty five per cent of the doctors had problems that could have been identified and treated during their student years.[8]

Again

> Medicine becomes a strain only when the physician asks himself to give more than he has been given. The long hours, the demanding patients, the ready access to narcotics were not a problem to the doctor whose childhood had been happy and who appeared psychologically sound by the time he reached college. Similarly a doctor

from an unhappy childhood may gain comfort and strength from
appreciative patients ... it is when the physician from a barren
childhood becomes overly burdened by the demands of his dependent patients that trouble arises. He, not the literally overworked
doctor, resorts to drugs to alleviate fatigue ... it was not the
physician who worked late who got divorced. But some physicians
worked late in response to unhappy marriages.[9]

There is a paradox in these conclusions: the doctors from
unhappy backgrounds may be weakened in their ability to
cope with the strains of professional life, but the selfsame
backgrounds may render them more sensitive to the needs of
their patients.

Some investigators have taken the question of the importance of early experiences one stage further by predicting
which medical students will eventually commit suicide[22]. In a
longitudinal survey of 1198 students at Johns Hopkins
medical school set up for 'precursors of hypertension and
coronary disease' it was found that between one and 18 years
after graduating, nine had committed suicide. For the
purpose of their 'retrospective–prospective' inquiry they
matched each of these nine with two controls from the larger
survey, plus six 'distractors' who included two who had died
'under ambiguous circumstances'. Information which was
available during the student years (early medical and family
history, academic record, smoking and drinking habits,
results of various psychological tests) relating to these 33
subjects was then shown blind to an investigator who had no
knowledge of their progress since qualification and who
arranged them in rank order for what was called their 'suicide
potential'. The first nine places in the rank were occupied by
the nine who had committed suicide.

Results such as these can seem extra-impressive to those
unfamiliar with studies on human behaviour, but nothing
concerning human behaviour can ever be explained
conclusively: at best a study like this can only give hints. Of
course, it is assumed at the outset by most workers in the
caring professions that early experiences have a profound
influence upon the quality of adult life and relationships, so
it is not surprising if these factors are emphasized. There is
nothing that can be done to change early experiences

although insights may be gained which may help avoid perpetuating problems, and medical schools could never possibly
exclude all candidates from unhappy backgrounds. But it
can be recognized that learning and practising medicine
impose emotional strains, and that it is nothing shameful for
a doctor to stumble or even to break down under the burden.
Because doctors are in the caring business, no one cares for
them, but then so many of them do make it impossibly
difficult for anyone, medical or non-medical, to see them as
live human beings with human weaknesses alongside all that
confidence and calm.

Doctors' wives

The wives of clergymen, lawyers, businessmen, politicians,
and many others may ask: what is so special about the
doctor's wife? They feel they too have hard lives, husbands
who have deep emotional commitments to their work,
irregular hours with meals delayed and social engagements
cancelled at the last moment, the privacy of the home
invaded by telephone calls or urgent knocks on the door, and
never being able to repel what come to seem like malevolent
intruders. They too may feel some sort of obligation to live
up to their husband's position, to affect a style of dress, to
espouse views, or to keep company that somehow sets him in
a favourable light.

They also may squirm inwardly when they hear praises of
their husband's kindness and patience, or of his unstinting
devotion to the welfare of others, of his ability to have time
for everyone despite his awesome responsibilities, and of
their great good fortune in being married to such a man.

However, it is the doctor's wife who seems to get the
greatest credit for her hard lot. Furthermore, she has
attracted a modest medical literature about herself which
seems to me to imply that she has a special role in our
society, has unique hardships to bear, and is at extra risk of
breaking down under the strain. For some reason a large
proportion of this literature comes from Canada.[23-26]

A study of fifty doctors' wives who required psychiatric
in-patient care revealed a good deal of distress: dissatisfaction with husbands who were described variously as

'undemonstrative, cold, dependent, domineering, perfection-
istic'; sexual problems and feelings of being excluded from
their husbands' work. They were women of all ages, and
presented mainly with depressive or anxiety symptoms.[27] In
other words they were like any group of married women
psychiatric patients from a professional background, and it
is only when drug-taking is considered that differences from
the expected emerge. (Other studies of doctors' wives also
found a high incidence of drug abuse.)[24,28]

Twenty-two of these 50 doctors' wives had problems with
drug-taking, and 11 of these were regarded as being addicted.
More detailed information was available for 16 of them, and
12 had obtained the drugs from their husbands' medical
supplies, with the husbands either administering the drugs
personally or else turning a blind eye to their use. Thirteen
of them had a complaint of pain, and some had had operative
procedures for pain during which time the drug taking began.

Independently of drug-taking, 21 had chronic pains of
various kinds, and the author suggests that there may be a
special angle to such complaints in a medical family. Pain is
a prime symptom which will engage the doctor's attention,
but the doctor then goes on to become frustrated when he
can find no explanation for the pain. In this way the
unhappy, and, it is implied, neglected wife successfully
demands from her husband the attention she supposes he
lavishes upon his patients. She then perpetuates this attention
and perhaps also punishes him a little by keeping him
guessing about the origin of the pain.

A reciprocal aspect of this theme is hinted at by a number
of the writers on doctors' ailments. Not only may some
women get themselves into a passive dependent, patient-like
relationship with their medical husbands, but the doctors
may find that the kind of relationship which suits them best
is the one they have with patients. They prefer to be
dominant at all times, and perhaps can only tolerate people
close to them provided those people occupy a subordinate
and acquiescent role. In other words, when they marry they
will marry someone who can occupy a patient role, but
patients will tend to have symptoms.

Doctors, like other professional people, usually marry

before they have realized their full potential. The medical
student and nurse are almost on a level before qualification,
and can work as close colleagues during the junior years, but
after that a gulf can develop. The gulf, which is seen by
psychiatrists dealing with marital problems amongst all
kinds of professional people not just doctors, is not so much
one of intellectual development but of attitude. The professional man has to develop his rational and practical functions,
while the wife, if she has children, evolves more on the
feeling level. If the husband is an authoritarian type with a
need to dominate, he will feel more comfortable with his
rational side where everything is predictable and controllable.
He will also find companions who can connect with this
rational side, and through it perhaps to his own less well
developed faculty for making a feeling relationship. The once
closely matched couple can easily get onto ever-diverging
courses where every event serves to accelerate the divergence.

Doctor's wife as housekeeper or partner

John Abernethy, surgeon and pupil of John Hunter, is
reported when he paid his last visit to a dying widow to have
taken her only daughter to one side and said:

> I have witnessed your devotion and kindness to your mother. I am in
> need of a wife, and I think you are the very person that would suit
> me. My time is incessantly occupied, and I have therefore no leisure
> for courting. Reflect upon this matter until Monday.[25]

She evidently accepted him, but in the 18th century an
unmarried woman on her own would have had little real
choice in the matter. Nevertheless, the story rings true of
attitudes to marriage (certainly of male attitudes) before
questions of 'relationship' and 'compatibility' predominated,
as they do now.

Around the end of the nineteenth century, Sir William
Osler was to offer advice probably typical of the age, in a
letter to a young doctor about to marry.

> There must be trust, gentleness and consideration. A doctor needs
> a woman who will look after his house and rear his children, a
> Martha whose first care will be for the home. Make her feel she is

your partner arranging a side of the business in which she should
have her sway and her way . . . console her and take her advice about
the house and children and keep to yourself as far as possible the
outside affairs relating to practice.[29]

Then, in an address to students:

What about the wife and babies, if you have them? Leave them!
Heavy as are your responsibilities to those nearest and dearest,
they are outweighed by the responsibilities to yourself, to the
profession, and to the public . . . Your wife will be glad to bear
her share in the sacrifice you make.[30]

These passages are redolent of paternalism and mystique
about the medical profession, and Sir William would be
saddened to see how the special status of doctors has
declined. Nevertheless they still have great authority over
other people in the course of clinical work. They do have a
greater immediate power than any of the other professionals
mentioned earlier, and it is a good working assumption that
some of this spills over into attitudes within the home.

Today there are a number of variations of the patterns of
involvement with, or separateness from, the medical
husband's occupation. Most wives have the educational background to comprehend their husband's work and they may
be closely involved in a practical way, even as medical
partners. Alternatively they may develop a way of partici-
pating in the problems and conflicts with a good
understanding of the issues yet personally remaining in the
background.

Some wives will elect for a more separate role. While they
are having children they may be exclusively orientated
towards the home, and may or may not develop outside
interests later. Others will have clear directions of their own,
in the form of major personal interests or else a different
career altogether.

No one can say which is the best of these styles, because
what matters is that the husband and wife remain in contact
at a feeling and a rational level. I know of no evidence to
suggest that wives who are involved in a real partnership with
their husbands fare better with regard to marital problems
than those who remain separate. Each style has its
advantages according to each individual's capacity for

emotional and intellectual development, but most people are deeply committed to married life before they experience the effects of such developmental dissonance. The conscious acceptance of such disparity between intellectual progress and intellectual stagnation on one hand, and between emotional blossoming and emotional stunting on the other, can be difficult and painful for most people, perhaps especially when it is the wife who has outdistanced the husband, but it is a necessary prerequisite for any real resolution of conflicts.

Women doctors

Most of this book derives from the activities of male doctors, and so it is inevitably written from a male standpoint: if over the past hundred years half the world's doctors had been women the book would have taken a different form.

About one-third of medical students and junior doctors are now women but they still have to compete in a male preserve, besides having had to compete harder to gain entry to medical school in the first place. They have had to develop their logical and intellectual functions to get themselves through the medical course but at the end of it they should represent the contemporary ideal of the liberated woman with high status and earning potential. The trouble is that at the end of the course they often see a career in medicine as making ever more demands on their intellectual qualities, when what they so often want to do is to be fulfilled in the more traditional women's roles. However, after years of study, accomplishment and responsibility this can be a difficult, even threatening, change of direction. It is as though the empathic or traditional feminine aspects of their nature were demanding an outlet but that the years of intellectual endeavour had made them less confident of the validity of their own feelings. This together with a sense of obligation to go on contributing to the medical care of the community and otherwise to make use of the education they have been given can be a painful dilemma to young women doctors.[31]   However, most of the trouble is in the anticipation, for women doctors seem to do as well as any other women in their maternal roles, and when the time comes to resume professional work they have better opportunities than most members of their sex.

Summary

Most people need some kind of mask before they can face the world in their professional capacity, and for doctors this mask fulfils the dual role of boosting self-esteem and acting as protective armour. In private, doctors are revealed to have high rates for psychosocial problems such as manifest psychological symptoms, marital problems and divorce, regular consultations with a psychiatrist, alcoholism and drug abuse and suicide. Some of the reasons for these difficulties are discussed, together with the predicaments of doctors' wives, and also of women doctors.

13. Fallibilities of Doctors

Doctors observe, make judgments and take action. Doctors are human, therefore they are fallible and liable to make errors without even realizing that anything is amiss.

Observer error

It seems that whenever two or more people study the same object different conclusions are reached about what is actually there.[1-3]

Take something definite life a chest X-ray film. Two radiologists and three chest specialists from different centres in the United States each reported on 1256 chest X-ray films as to whether they were positive or negative for tuberculosis. The number of positive reports given by the five readers varied between 56 and 100. 'In some cases . . . 20 per cent of the films called positive for tuberculosis by one reader were called negative by another'. The five readers were then given a second look at the 1256 films. One who had picked out 59 positives on his first reading found 78 positive on the second.[4]

In another survey in which six readers studied 150 pairs of X-ray films taken about three months apart, the authors concluded:

> in judging a pair of films for evidence of progression, regression, or stability of disease in patients with pulmonary tuberculosis, two readers are likely to disagree with each other in almost one-third of

the cases and a single reader is likely to contradict himself in approximately one fifth of cases.[5]

Although far more direct clinical observations are made on
patients than on the results of laboratory or X-ray investigations, there are relatively few studies on observer error in
the clinical field. However, those that have been done all tell
the same story. Surgeons at the Leeds Department of
Surgery[6] investigated the performance of three independent
clinicians with eight patients with 'severe, acute attacks of
ulcerative colitis'.

They compared the agreement amongst the three clinicians
with the agreement which might be expected by chance. With
regard to the

> presence of tenderness, rebound tenderness or distension, the
> severity of tenderness, overall clinical status, and management
> recommendations . . . the degree of agreement was at least twice that
> expected by chance . . . [but] other aspects of the clinical exam-
> ination of these patients . . . were less satisfactory. The observer
> agreement concerning guarding of the abdominal musculature and
> concerning the findings on percussion of the abdomen was roughly
> that which might have been obtained by chance . . . in nearly half of
> the total assessments the three observers were unable to agree among
> themselves whether the patient was getting better or worse . . .
> Finally, there were some aspects of the clinical examination of these
> patients in which the instances of agreement between the observers
> were so infrequent as to render them of little practical value. For
> example, in only 8.3 per cent of the assessments was it agreed that
> the patient looked pale, a proportion of agreement which is less
> than that expected by chance. In 2.8 per cent of the assessments it
> was agreed that the patient appeared anaemic . . . The mean haemo-
> globin level of these patients was just over 70 per cent on admission.

Agreement on the presence or absence of dehydration or muscular rigidity was never reached at all. The authors conclude:

> This poor evaluation of the clinical picture was obtained in spite of
> ready availability of biochemical data to all three observers, and
> despite the provision at each assessment of a detailed data chart
> concerning the patient's symptoms, temperature, pulse rate, and
> stools during the 12 hours before each assessment.

They wonder whether ulcerative colitis is a 'special case' but
this report is in full agreement with other similar studies. In
fact this universal agreement about the unreliability of
human observation is the only unanimous finding to emerge.

Of course accurate observation is impossible and no true description can ever be given of the natural world. At best there can only be an approximation — a fact well known to physical scientists. For doctors the problem is further compounded by both subject and object being fallible, emotional and unpredictable humans, so that the best any doctor can do is to be conscious of the limitations of the processes and the kinds of factors which can mislead him.

General physical and mental state

Clinical efficiency, or any other kind of activity calling for high levels of vigilance and decision making, can be seriously impaired by long hours of activity, and good physical and mental health is no protection. Lack of sleep is the most obvious factor, but the general level of anxiety can aggravate the effects of sleep loss or else precipitate adverse reactions in the apparently well rested.

Sleep loss. Extensive laboratory testing of subjects deprived of sleep shows that a measurable deterioration in performance can be reliably demonstrated after one night with only two hours sleep, or after two consecutive nights with only five hours slept on each.[7] Where one whole night has been spent without any sleep at all, performance is much more seriously impaired, and even one good night's sleep is not sufficient to restore the subject to full efficiency. These findings were based on inevitably dull tests of vigilance, and if subjects are engaged in activities which are inherently interesting or, better still, vitally important, their performance will be less affected by sleep loss.[8]

One of the first effects of tiredness in actual practice is slowing down; the making of mistakes generally comes later. Hospital doctors feel they are chronically short of sleep, and this matter was investigated by a group at the Presbyterian Hospital, New York City.[9] Fourteen interns (13 men and 1 woman) were tested when well rested and again when deprived of sleep in the course of the night-time duties. On each occasion they completed rating scales dealing with mood variables, and another dealing with 'psychophysiological' factors. Also they had to read an electrocardiograph tracing and indicate the episodes showing abnormalities of rhythm.

In their rested state they had had on average 7 hours of sleep, when fatigued on average 1.8 hours (range 0–3.8 hours). When rested they made an average of 5.2 errors in interpreting the electrocardiograph tracing (prizes of $50 and $25 were offered for the fewest errors made in the reporting when tired), and 9.6 when sleep-deprived. The mood scale showed significantly less 'vigor, elation, and social affection', and significantly more 'fatigue and sadness'. In the psychophysiological scale they made significantly more complaints such as feeling weak or nauseated or having difficulty in focussing their eyes.

Four of the 14 stopped the electrocardiograph during the experimental and control trials, and three of these four took on average 7.3 minutes longer to complete their study of the record when fatigued than when rested although this extra time did not seem to improve their performance.

The message from such studies is that although a doctor may *appear* to be doing his job adequately after many hours or even days without proper sleep, it should not be assumed that he is really coping. He is probably working at an almost subconscious level, and any change from well practised routines might be disastrous.

Anxiety level. A certain amount of anxiety can be a good thing. A junior doctor, unsure of his ability to cope with all eventualities, may be stimulated to take extra care over everything he does. Unfortunately, the dividing line between what is a stimulating challenge and what is demoralising, frustrating and overwhelming is hard to draw. Also, what may be stimulating in the short term can prove unmanageable if it has to be endured for a long period.

Surgeons, and others who carry out physical procedures on patients, can sometimes become highly anxious if, for example, a clamp slips off a large vessel, if stitches keep tearing out of friable gut, if the common bile duct is thought to have been cut at the bottom of a deep fat-lined hole and proper exposure is impossible. These are circumstances which can give the doctor momentary feelings of panic that he will lose control of the situation and the patient will die while he stands by helpless. It is just at such moments, especially if the doctor concerned is also tired, that a faulty interpretation of the event may lead to precipitate action which could have catastrophic results.

More important even are the extraneous anxieties and concerns. Everybody lives with conflict in some degree: there may be simple disagreements at work about the allocation of resources or there may be painful personal disputes with colleagues. At home, there may be matrimonial difficulties, and perhaps a deep-seated on-going conflict between responsibility to work and responsibility to home and family. These personal problems, partly because they involve emotions and partly because they are in their nature ill-defined and have no simple correct solution, may at times threaten to upset the doctor's calm clinical appraisal and judgment.

Adverse reactions[10-12]

Poor concentration, forgetfulness, and elementary mistakes. This is an early stage in fatigue which with experience subjects can come to recognize in themselves. Everything slows down and there is a tendency to check details over and over again, so that an abdominal examination normally taking one minute is greatly extended, and with several return visits to the patient to make quite sure that nothing has been overlooked. Things are put down somewhere, and then cannot be found. There is a tendency to be irritable, or alternatively to be excessively relaxed and phlegmatic.

Shock, apathy, and the inability to act. Certain medical catastrophes can render the best organized doctor at least temporarily paralysed and inarticulate — the sudden arrival in a casualty department of a dozen patients with severe multiple injuries, a massive haemorrhage from an unknown source, total disruption of an abdominal wound. All these can be quite bewildering to the tired or hard-pressed doctor.

A period of apathetic inability to do anything may be inevitable, and it should be accepted for it is much preferable to useless activity; the weary doctor will gradually organize his thoughts and decide where his first efforts should be directed.

Panic, useless activity and compounding errors. Although it is extremely unlikely that a doctor will panic completely in the face of an emergency, there are extreme circumstances which will occur from time to time. In disasters, especially where there is a personal involvement such as someone's own child being trapped in the wreckage, there are examples of doctors clawing uselessly at the rubble when they ought to have been at their medical base; or else of doctors so overwhelmed by the events that their behaviour becomes quite disorganized and they dab ineffectually or even suture up infected wounds.[13,14]

Another kind of panic reaction can occur after one error has been made. It is probably realized that something is wrong but instead of taking corrective action the error is repeated, and each successive act aggravates the crisis rather than alleviating it. Every surgeon is at risk of doing this. He mistakenly makes too large a cut during his dissection, but instead of retreating (or even being frozen briefly into inactivity) he makes another cut, and yet another until he has a major problem on his hands. The same kind of thing seems to occur in road, rail and air accidents. An error is made — acceleration instead of braking. The fatigued driver (from tiredness and/or anxiety) may not correct the mistake by braking firmly but may accelerate more, sometimes with fatal results.[12]

False expectations. The surgeon is roused from his bed in the middle of the night to see what he rapidly assumes to be a case of acute appendicitis. Other clinical features which do not conform to this expectation are ignored. (Of course this can happen any time as discussed in Chapter 3 but the consequences may be more dramatic when the doctor is fatigued.) Even at operation the significance of the circulatory collapse and grossly distended gut may not be grasped, and the fatigued surgeon may grope around for a while inside the abdominal cavity seemingly unable to comprehend what is already obvious to his assistants — that the patient is suffering from acute intestinal obstruction. It is an example of seeing what one would like to see rather than what is actually there and, once having reached a conclusion (however erroneous), of being extremely slow to modify it despite the insistent evidence. The simple truth has to be pointed out by somebody else.

Preoccupation and distraction. In the early days of cardiac resuscitation I once saw a registrar so unnerved by a cardiac arrest that he threw himself into the business of getting a blood transfusion going, which he insisted on doing as an essential preliminary to cardiac massage, despite the objections of the rest of us. He was concentrating on an activity which he could understand when faced with a larger problem which was beyond him, but, more importantly and dangerously, he had re-interpreted the problem of cardiac arrest to suit his limitations, and nothing anyone could do at the time could shift him in his beliefs.

Unfortunately the danger is not over just because the immediate crisis has passed. Indeed the time for greatest vigilance can be just that time when it seems that everyone can relax. This *relaxation after stress* can lead the surgeon to take insufficient care in suturing up the wound at the end of a difficult operation, or it can cause him to be less than thorough over the next emergency case he has to see, and lead him possibly to a diagnosis favouring inaction, and so an earlier return to bed. The slightly weary, benevolent feeling that can come over doctors after any late-night emergency acitivity can, I suspect, contain a false sense of self-confidence if there are other emergency cases to be seen.

Assumptions and beliefs

It is not possible simply to 'observe'. If a class of students were told to 'observe', and to write down what they had observed, they would have no idea where to begin because before any observation is possible there must be certain assumptions about what is to be looked for, and certain restrictions because the amount of information in any scene is for practical purposes infinite.[15] Doctors, for example, make the assumption that the person they have been called to see may be ill, and that illness may manifest itself by certain phenomena they call symptoms and physical signs.

Doctors, like the judiciary, have an incorrigible habit of embellishing their observations with moral judgments, and this further clouds the accuracy of their perceptions. Alex Comfort[16] has chronicled the deplorable behaviour of the medical profession in this respect. His account of the extreme attitudes taken by high-minded doctors in the past reads like fantasy nowadays, but is not. The preposterous attitudes taken up publicly by doctors on matters like masturbation, contraception, artificial insemination, not to mention their equally high-minded advocacy of barbarous and unproven remedies, were a painful reality to the helpless patients who were made to endure a totally unnecessary sense of guilt.

No subject better exemplifies the moral presumption of the medical profession than its preoccupation with the supposed evils of masturbation culminating in the notion of 'masturbatory insanity'. The fact that papers on the subject appeared in the *Lancet* in the nineteenth century indicates that these were not the utterances of isolated cranks but that they reflected ideas currently acceptable to the profession as a whole.[17,18] Now, masturbation is no longer regarded in that light, but that is the way with 'authoritarian' attitudes: prejudices and values will change according to the dictates of established authority. In this case, of course, the authority was the medical profession itself, but I suspect a change had to come imperceptibly from the leaders of the profession in view of the fact that no real evidence ever emerged to support the concept of masturbatory insanity. Other prejudices were found to take its place.

At the beginning of the twentieth century when masturbation was starting to lose its grip on the medical imagination, the evils of coffee- and tea-drinking were being discovered. Around this time the Regius Professor of Physic at Cambridge along with the most distinguished pharmacologist of the time described in a standard medical textbook the effects of excessive coffee consumption: 'the sufferer is tremulous and loses his self-command; he is subject to fits of agitation and depression.' Tea was no better: 'producing nightmares with . . . hallucinations which may be alarming in their intensity . . . [and] a strange and extreme degree of physical depression . . so that . . the speech may become weak and vague'.[19]

This passage (which would have served quite well a few decades earlier as a description of the consequences of masturbation) was quoted from a British government inquiry into the use of cannabis. Around the time the passage was written cannabis was in the pharmacopoeia, and the benefits of mescaline were being reported in the medical press.[20,21] In the 1960s and early 1970s cannabis was the evil, and coffee and tea socially acceptable.

Despite several years of intensive study cannabis has not been seriously incriminated, and so the quasi-scientific literature[22] is drying up and the severity of court sentences has declined. But what will the medical profession latch on to next?

Abortion is a topic which divides opinion sharply and generates plenty of feeling. Those strongly 'for' or 'against' abortion will base their emotive arguments on supposedly rational grounds, and each side will read the literature to suit what I would regard as its emotional position. The great mistake and misdemeanour that the doctors are making is in offering their prejudices or moral views as empirical medical truth. Doctors have a right to moral values like everybody else but they must learn to become conscious of their moral position on all topics relevant to clinical medicine. They should also take on the harder task of learning to become sensitive to their prejudices (mentioned in Chapter 3) as evidenced, for example, by the experience of powerful antagonism or anxiety in a routine clinical situation.

Sometimes the medical profession gives advice which is frankly irrational. Why else would doctors throughout the English-speaking world recommend circumcision in the absence of clinical indications or religious requirement[23,24,25]

Summary

Human fallibilities damage the conception of clinical medicine as an exact science. The simplest observation is fraught with potential errors. Tiredness and/or anxieties (connected with the doctor's work or in his private life) may seriously impair the reliability of his judgment, sometimes with disastrous consequences. The doctor's personal beliefs and prejudices can also exert a powerful influence on his clinical judgment, so he must try to become conscious of these factors and allow for them.

14. The Wounded Physician

The need to be a doctor

To the outsider, medicine is the ideal answer to the perennial dilemma of trying to find a life with meaning. Non-medical people are forever telling doctors how they have often thought of taking up medicine themselves, and how utterly worthwhile it must be to be doing good for so many people. The clergy speak half-enviously to doctors about being able to do real practical good for people, and not just attending to their souls, as they put it. Doctors take this kind of talk for granted, and bask in it a little for it makes them feel comfortable. Alongside their complaints about the organization of medical services and what they see as their generally hard lot in society, where they feel they are either underpaid or else adequately rewarded but impossibly hard-pressed, few doctors stop to think that they may actually practise medicine because they have a personal need to do so. Whatever may have motivated a young person to take up the study of medicine in the first place, clinical practice becomes the chosen field because being there face to face with patients actually does the doctor a great deal of good.

Few ideas could be farther from the consciousness of the modern doctor than the idea that his patients are meeting some needs of his. He is, after all, the rock on whom they can rely in their travail. He has the knowledge, the experience and the facilities to bring about a cure and remove the evil of illness. Amid all the dread of threatening illness, the doctor alone is confident. Indeed he is dependable and self-sufficient in the best traditions of Western protestantism, and has

176

justly earned for himself the love and respect of the community. How could such a rock-like figure have needs which are met by the sick and the weak? How indeed, yet what would he be without them?

A number of writers have referred to an apparent need of doctors to care for others (see Chapter 12 on sick and troubled doctors). In some cases it is a desire to look after people, in others a more specific need to give to others the love and attention that had never been experienced in the doctor's own childhood. At first sight this would seem to be wholly desirable, as in competitive societies few enough people may seem to care for anything but their own interest. Unfortunately, however, caring is not a simple matter of one person doing good for another. There is a negative side to caring as there is a negative, or dark, or simply reverse side to everything that happens or that people do. A mother's love is always taken as the prime example of selfless giving, and it can come as a shock to discover that mothers can be destructive as well as supportive: it is not for nothing that the vulture is one of the ancient symbols for the mother.[1]

The dividing line between genuine caring and damaging possessiveness or over-protectiveness is hard to define but the consequences of such destructive relationships are clearly recognizable.[2] It is much less clear when doctors themselves fall unwittingly into these interpersonal traps.

Whenever someone may be deriving personal sustenance from his work and surroundings, there will be an emotional investment, and that means that there is bound to be a danger of extra emotion causing undesirable responses. As far as doctors are concerned certain aspects of this problem have already been mentioned: the need to keep others dependent and only allow people close if they adopt a submissive (patient-like) manner, the development of an unhealthy yearning for power, the tendency to pass emotive moralizing judgments on patients.

Magician to technologist: the evolution of the modern doctor

In ancient societies with a world-view which interpreted human misfortune, and so many other events, in terms of the action of supernatural forces, the priest and the healer had closely related and overlapping roles. Both were the agents of the supernatural forces, and in dealing with the sick the emphasis was on the process of healing because in those times there was no body of empirical knowledge such as would be necessary before there could be anything resembling the practice of medicine as it would be understood today.

Who the first empirical practitioners were is not known. The Egyptians seem to have made a start a very long time ago, but for the present purposes it is convenient to begin with Hippocrates because he was the first to leave behind a systematic body of work and one which is still readily intelligible in principle twenty-five centuries later. His main contribution was in establishing that

> disease was a natural process, that its symptoms were the reactions of the body to the disease, and that the chief function of the physician was to aid the natural forces of the body.[3]

The idea that disease is a natural process as opposed to a supernatural one is taken for granted in the modern world. The idea that the function of the physician is to aid the natural forces of the body would be seen from the modern point of view as a hopeful rationalization of doctors who, clever as they might have been, had few remedies at their disposal. Yet this idea contained elements of importance which have become obscured by the brilliant success of technological medicine. They can be better understood by reference to the *cult of Asclepius* which flourished on the island of Cos alongside the Hippocratic school.

This was a priestly cult working in the name of Apollo, 'the god who kills, yet purifies and heals'.[4] There were temples in various parts of ancient Greece in healthy sites with pure spring water such as might be selected nowadays for a spa or a health resort, and the most famous of these was at Epidauros. The sick person would come to the sanctuary not to see a doctor who would administer treatment, but rather to encounter directly the powers of healing. Not the kind of healing that might be expected or hoped for as a result of prayer or an offering to a deity, but one regarded as having been activated by the healing powers felt to be latent within each person. To achieve this the patient would withdraw to the innermost chamber of the sanctuary, and there rest. In the deep sleep that followed the patient dreamed or experienced healing visions. He had withdrawn from the priestly physicians and surrendered himself to whatever powers he could summon from within his being.[4] There is nothing magical about this, and the idea that each person has a potential for healing present within himself — in addition to the efforts of the doctors — represented a spiritual aspect which blended well with the more practical disciplines of the Hippocratic workers. Hippocrates was well established on the island of Cos before the Asclepians arrived there (although the original priestly cult had been in existence for a long time) but the Hippocratic oath opens with a reference to them: 'I swear by Apollo the physician, and Asclepius, and Hygeia and Panacea [Asclepius' daughters] . . . '

Here then is a dual approach to the care of the sick: on one hand empirically derived knowledge is used to relieve symptoms or to influence known disease processes, and on the other whatever powers of self-healing the individual may possess are simultaneously activated.

In mediaeval Europe the sick were cared for by the monastic orders where knowledge from the ancient world was kept alive, although illness itself tended to be seen as a punishment for sinfulness. With the coming of the renaissance, secular medical schools were established in different parts of Europe, and also organizations for the regulation of medical practice. Nevertheless, the religious tradition was strong insofar as it influenced the personal attitudes of the practitioners of medicine, and perhaps its best aspects can be summarized by the famour words of Ambroise Pare (1510–90): 'I dressed him; God healed him'. There was also the alchemical tradition which in its essence was concerned with spiritual exploration, and could serve to connect doctors with the supra-rational.

When the new enlightenment dawned, there was a doctor in at the beginning. He was William Harvey (1578–1657) and his discovery of the circulation of the blood perfectly matched the ideas about scientific method of Francis Bacon (1561–1626) and the mechanistic views of Descartes (1596–

1650). However, God was still central in the intellectual systems of these people and was to remain so for some time yet. Both Locke (1632–1714), who was a distinguished doctor as well as an empiricist philosopher, and Newton (1642–1727) went to great lengths to reconcile their empirical scientific activities with their religion; and Newton always regarded his religious and alchemical writings as more important than his mathematical and scientific contributions.

After their time, with medicine now well established as an independent profession and discoveries coming along at an increasing rate, less and less was heard about ideas of healing. That is not to say that people were any less religious, simply that the emphasis was now on the practical issue of what could be done to relieve the sick, which of course was admirable. There must have been great excitement then (as there has been at all times since when whole new areas of knowledge seem to be opening up) at the possibilities ahead, and it was quite right that the effort should go outward and into the practical world. Doctors were becoming more central figures in the community, and so began to identify with the material values of the society they were serving. This trend further increased the emphasis on the practical and away from what might have been regarded in the past as the priestly functions, and the pattern still exists today.

In the latter part of the twentieth century there is an increasing awareness among medical workers of the importance of psychosocial factors but medical ideas about healing are still purely mechanistic. Outside of medicine, however, there is a great interest in questions of healing, as of course there always has been. Faith healers, religious groups conducting healing rituals, and all kinds of fringe medical activities have concentrated on the healing processes without much reference to the actual disease they are trying to eliminate. It is this latter approach which characterized the Asclepians insofar as it recognizes that the patient himself has a part to play in the healing process. It is not enough simply to attack the disease, because, as has been shown throughout this book, the personality, emotions and lifestyle of the patient all affect the outcome. It is the whole person who must be taken into account. The word 'healing' means 'making whole'.

Psychotherapy as a paradigm of medical practice

The more complicated and more powerful the medical machine becomes, the less can the average patient participate actively in what is going on; indeed nothing is asked of the patient except passive compliance. Furthermore, medicine — especially in its wider social context — is now being practised more anonymously than it used to be. Intimate case records are housed in large centres where all members of staff of the organization concerned have *de facto* access to them, and there is talk of getting the entire medical record into data retrieval systems. Against this background the patient becomes less of an individual, and also — which is the point at issue here — less able to participate in his own cure.

For that reason the psychotherapeutic interview is being taken as an example of doctor and patient meeting in a professional context where their interaction is not encumbered by the presence of organic illness, hospitalization, drug treatment or surgical operation. Although there may be no overt illness there is often much more sheer distress and misery than is generated as a result of the majority of physical illnesses.

There is an assumption in this encounter that the patient's difficulties have arisen not as a result of a disease process, but rather as a result of the patient's own inability (for a great variety of reasons) to cope with his present circumstances in life. Therefore the therapist is not going to try to *do* things to the patient in the sense that most doctors do, rather he is going to try to help the patient to gain insights into his difficulties so that the patient essentially will be able to find his own way out of those difficulties.

The essential ingredients of the psychotherapeutic process are first, knowledge on the part of the therapist about human behaviour and the vagaries of mental functioning, and secondly, a secure yet challenging relationship in which the troubled patient can explore and work upon his problems. Of the two, the second is the more important for the purposes of the present discussion.

The patient is distressed and perplexed by his problems. He knows well enough that trouble exists, but he has little understanding of its essential nature or why he is so afflicted. Still less, has he any idea what to do about it.

Any exploration of one's private self is likely at the outset to involve a good deal of pain. That is, the recognition and frank acceptance of a great deal within which is bad, shameful or otherwise contrary to the conscious feeling of what one would like to be. If physical illness is the issue, instead of psychological distress, then there has to be an acceptance of the reality of the illness. There must be an acceptance that this is one's own illness, that it is part of one's self, because that is undeniably what it is. Even if the illness was the direct result of some outside agent or an accident, the condition is still the patient's and nobody else's. So many people speak of their illness as though it was not part of them, rather it is seen as some alien influence which must be eliminated. However, the patient who either has the innate ability to meet these realities on his own, or else has a doctor who will sustain him while he struggles towards them, has the capacity to bring a great deal of constructive mental energy to bear on to the business of getting better, and will, I suspect, be the one who makes the best recovery, or who recovers or survives against the odds.

The idea that each patient has a positive part to play in his illness, and contains within himself a potential for healing has been expressed by some writers in terms of: 'the healer within the patient'.[5] Therefore instead of saying of the patient who appears to have no will to recover: 'this patient does not want to get well', one might say 'this patient has not been able to draw on the healing potential within himself'.

Demands on the doctor

Although some degree of need to care is probably a requirement for a clinician, that very need which can cause him to be so supportive can also lead him astray. The cumulative load of the emotional input from all the patients is familiar to those in psychotherapeutic practice but is present in all clinical encounters whether it is explicitly acknowledged or not.

The doctor—patient interaction is a two-way affair, and the doctor's feelings about the patient also have to be acknowledged. The doctor is perfectly well able to recognize the patient's emotional responses, although when they are flattering to him he may well fail to recognize them for what they really are. However it is the doctor's responses which are of the greater importance because, apart from anything else, there can be no one regularly at hand to point out his foibles to him. The pychotherapist face to face with a series of individual patients is especially prone to these difficulties. In some cases his patients may suffer as a result or simply fail to benefit as much as they ought to, but more serious in the long run are the dangers to the doctor.[5]

Some of the harmful consequences of the great power and prestige that doctors enjoy have been discussed in Chapter 11, The Honoured Practitioner, and it was suggested that these might arise because of difficulties the doctor experienced in the course of clinical work. The doctor has demands made on him which made him feel uncomfortable but which he is generally unable to recognize for what they are — the emotional tensions consequent upon the close relationship between two people, doctor and patient. One way of dealing with this ill-understood discomfort is to avoid those circumstances where doctor and patient can face one another on equal terms, or else to develop a style of working which keeps patients at a safe distance.

The doctor thus avoids that part of his clinical practice which could be called 'caring' as opposed to 'treating'. He deprives himself of a kind of satisfaction which he probably needs, and is certainly not likely to be fulfilled by adopting more clinically remote or administrative roles.

The wounded healer

Some able clinicians who are held in high esteem by their colleagues may be scarcely noticed by the patients while some quite mediocre doctors can be almost revered in their practices.

When people (including doctors) are asked what they have thought of the doctor or dentist they have just seen, they are likely to give a fairly immediate and definite opinion. These people are seldom in a position to express a considered opinion of the professional worth of the practitioner concerned but they are able to recognize someone who relates to them and seems to care about them. In other words they are most likely to be expressing an opinion about the doctor's or the dentist's empathic qualities and other attributes peripheral to clinical skill. What these qualities are (and also how they may be learned if need be) is naturally an issue of some interest in psychotherapy, and there has certainly been plenty of research in that direction[6] but questions of feeling, and empathy and relationships are always liable to prove elusive to the investigator.

I would prefer not to try to chase those elusive attributes but to look more at the circumstances which favour their development, in particular *the idea of the wound*. It is epitomised in the statement: 'Only the wounded physician heals'. A curious notion perhaps to those who feel that the doctor should always be the secure rock, but I can illustrate the idea with a simple example. A professional man planned and carried out a theft of some articles from a shop. He was duly apprehended and brought to court. The sentence was nominal but a greater punishment for him was the fact that the deed was reported widely in the local and even in the national newspapers. He was publicly branded with having done the one thing a man in his position should never do: like a priest committing adultery, a doctor killing his patient, or a lawyer swindling a client. The prospect of returning to his work was shattering. He felt no one henceforward could have any respect for him, his word could no longer be trusted, and he expected to be abused by those who had formerly shown him respect — and he felt of course that their reactions would be entirely justified. What happened in fact was almost the reverse. While nobody dismissed or denied the seriousness of what had happened, there was friendship rather than abuse. People came forward with an openness and warmth that he had not experienced before. They said: 'Oh, I could never talk to you before'. Or 'I had been wanting to tell you this for a long time but couldn't. I feel I can now'. He found that people felt they could reveal themselves more honestly than before, as though because he had been shown to be less than perfect they could reveal and acknowledge that they too were less than perfect. This was not just a temporary phenomenon, it led to a much deeper degree of understanding with his colleagues, and led to enrichment in his personal life as well.

Most people, and certainly most professional people, find themselves wearing a mask. It is not usually of their conscious making but it provides a protection which is understandable. Sometimes the mask is shattered by an event, such as happened to the man just described, or in the case of someone who has a near-fatal illness, or any experience which leads to a fundamental reappraisal of values in life. A few people seem to go though life without the need for such armour, but what is common to all people who have either shed, or have never had, a protective mask is the idea of vulnerability. By laying down their armour they are declaring that they are not perfect and inviolable. Although perhaps not actually indicating their weaknesses, they are accepting the possibility of personal weakness, and it is that potential which other people can discern and relate to.

The idea of the value of the weakness — or the 'wound' as it can be called — is very old, particularly in regard to healing. Asclepius was taught his healing arts according to legend by Chiron, the centaur. Chiron suffered a wound (not specified to my knowledge) which would never heal, and this was judged necessary for him in his special role. Chiron was a divine figure in Greek mythology, and so his wound must be seen in a symbolic light, so that 'this mythological physician . . . embodied for men of later times . . . nothing other than the knowledge of a wound in which the healer forever partakes'.[4]

In many cultures it has been expected that the healer will also be a sufferer, and this is most vividly demonstrated in those societies where there are Shamans.[7,8] These are people regarded as having a mixture of priestly and healing powers, but a requirement for the role is that they should possess some defect such as in Western society would be recognized as an illness or disability, often of a spectacular kind such as epilepsy, although it would be expected that they had mastered the condition or else somehow come to terms with it. In their own cultures what might seem to Westerners as a weakness was seen as evidence of the ability to communicate with the spirit world, and thus was conceptualized in positive terms.

Shamanistic practices are rather extreme but in some degree the principle that the healer is also impaired will be found in many primitive and tribal societies. In the Christian culture the principle is exemplified in the person of Jesus. He was the healer, who had no power and no status in the community, so that in temporal terms he was ineffectual. He was important in his lifetime to those who had known him directly, but his world-wide influence was to begin only after he had been betrayed, publicly humiliated, chastised, and put to death. Later, in words attributed to St Peter, it was expressed: 'By his wounds you have been healed'.[9] Peter himself had earlier denied even having known Jesus, and he had to carry that wound — that reminder for him of his human frailty — with him throughout his subsequent ministry.

What then is the relevance of these ideas to the contemporary practice of medicine? Is it necessary for every doctor to suffer before he can be deemed adequate to discharge the role of healer? Is the technological training to be augmented by a psychological or a spiritual one? There can be no answer for everyone. In the Christian culture it is sometimes assumed that suffering is a necessary prerequisite for real personal development but this is not necessarily assumed in the concept of the wounded healer. What is assumed, indeed demanded, is that the practitioner recognize (perhaps as Peter had been compelled to) the possibility that he is vulnerable. Every doctor knows, of course, that he is as prone, if not more prone, to illness as the next man but he does not act as though this was the case. So often his high status, his need for power and local distinction causes these human awarenesses to be pushed into the background so that the patient is left facing a shell of a person. An alcoholic doctor may be a public menace but he is a credible human because his wounds and weaknesses are plainly apparent, and so he may be approached in preference to the respectable citizen. But, it may be objected, the doctor ought to be above reproach. He should be someone of the highest integrity, not someone who is the victim of human weaknesses. Over the centuries professional standards have been tightened and raised by the influence of supervisory bodies. Through them the public has gained a great deal but something has also been lost.

Technologist or wounded healer

How is the doctor to reconcile the desire to enjoy the benefits of his position in society and the opportunities that derive from having a relatively high income, with the image of the healer who has one foot in weakness or even in madness? How is the technologically advanced doctor who has spent years acquiring specialized knowledge or refining his skills to justify spending hours with the distressed and the frightened? How could the members of a great profession think of learning from witch-doctors in primitive tribes?

The success of medical science over the past hundred years has engendered a passivity in the minds of the lay public which has flattered the doctors' sense of power and self-esteem. It has also caused people to assume less and less responsibility for what happens to their bodies and to their minds, and to ease doctors imperceptibly into the dangerous position where they privately come to believe that they can control everything.

The greatest benefit could come in the future if patients could take on more responsibility for their bodies and minds, in other words learn to activate the potential for help and healing that is latent within themselves. Doctors then may come to acknowledge, perhaps through a greater openness in their own lives, that they too are needy and vulnerable along with the patient, and that doctoring is something of a joint venture between patient and healer, in which the doctor serves as the guide.

Summary

Although the modern clinical doctor may like to see himself as the detached provider of technical expertise, I am suggesting that the doctor practises clinical medicine because such work fulfils a need in him. In the past the doctor was more of a mediator whose role was in part to help the sick person to make contact with the healing potential within himself. At the present time this approach is out of favour although psychotherpay provides an example of how the doctor and patient can work together with each making a contribution. Some kind of partnership between doctor and patient is desirable and possible in all branches of clinical medicine.

References

*indicates a reference to a review article or textbook.

Chapter 1: Meaning in illness

1   Planck, M. (1933) *Where is Science Going?* London: Allen and Unwin.

2   Bennet, G. (1974) Scientific medicine? *Lancet*, 2, 453–6.

3   Scadding, J.G. (1967) Diagnosis: the clinician and the computer. *Lancet*, 2, 877–81.

*4   Lusted, L.B. (1968) *Introduction to Medical Decision Making.* Springfield, Ill.: Charles C Thomas.

5   Williams, R.J. (1956) *Biochemical Individuality.* New York: John Wiley.

Chapter 2: Non-medical views of illness

*1   Tuckett, D. (ed) (1976) *An Introduction to Medical Sociology.* London: Tavistock Publications.

2   Parsons, T. (1951) *The Social System.* Chicago: The Free Press of Glencoe.

*3   Parkes, C.M. (1972) *Bereavement: Studies of Grief in Adult Life.* London: Tavistock Publications (Harmondsworth:Penguin).

*4   Dohrenwend, B.S. & Dohrenwend, B.P. (1974) *Stressful Life Events: Their Nature and Effects.* New York: Wiley.

5   Fried, M. Grieving for a lost home. Cited in (3).

6   Keddie, K.M.G. (1977) Pathological mourning after the death of a domestic pet. *Br. J. Psychiat.*, *131*, 21–5.

189

7 Parkes, C.M. (1975) Psycho-social transitions: Comparison between reactions to loss of a limb and loss of a spouse. *Br. J. Psychiat., 127,* 204—10.

8 Bennet, G. (1970) Bristol floods 1968: Controlled survey of effects on health of local community disaster. *Br. med. J., 3,* 454—8.

9 Lorraine, N.S.R. (1954) Canvey Island flood disaster, February 1953. *Med. Officer, 91* 59—62.

10 Hinkle, L.E. & Wolff, H.G. (1958) Ecologic investigations of the relationship between illness, life experiences and the social environment. *Ann. intern. Med., 49,* 1373—88.

11 Rahe, R.H., McKean, J.D. jun. & Arthur, R.J. (1967) A longitudinal study of life change and illness patterns. *J. psychosom. Res., 10,* 355—66.

*12 Gunderson, E.K.E. & Rahe, R.H. (eds) (1974) *Life Stress and Illness.* Springfield, Ill.: Charles C Thomas.

*13 Birley, J.L.T. & Connolly, J. (1976) Life events and physical illness. *Mod. Trends psychosom. Med., 3,* 154—65.

14 Schless, A.P., Teichman, A., Mendels, J., Weinstein, N.W. & Weller, K. (1977) Life events and illness: a three year prospective study. *Br. J. Psychiat., 131,* 26—34.

15 Theorell, T., Lind, E. & Flodérus, B. (1973) The relationship of disturbing life-changes and emotions to the early development of myocardial infarction and other serious illnesses. *Int. J. Epidemiol., 4,* 281—93.

*16 Lipowski, Z.J. (1976) Psychosomatic medicine: An overview. *Mod. Trends psychosom. Med., 3,* 1—20.

*17 Reiser, M.F. (1975) Changing theoretical concepts in psychosomatic medicine. In: *American Handbook of Psychiatry,* ed. S. Arieti, 2nd ed., vol. 4, pp. 477—500. New York: Basic Books.

18 Friedman, M. & Rosenman, R.H. (1959) Association of specific overt behaviour pattern with blood and cardiovascular findings. *J. Am. med. Ass., 169,* 1286—96.

19 Friedman, M. & Rosenman, R.H. (1974) *Type A Behaviour and Your Heart.* New York: Knopf (London: Wildwood House).

20 Rosenman, R.H., Brand, R.J., Jenkins, C.D., Friedman, M., Straus, R. & Wurm, M. (1975) Coronary heart disease in the Western collaborative group study: final follow-up of 8½ years. *J. Am. med. Ass., 233,* 872—7.

21 Rosenman, R.H. & Friedman, M. (1971) The central nervous system and coronary heart disease. *Hosp. Pract., 5,* 87—97.

*22 Groen, J.J. (1976) Psychosomatic aspects of ischaemic (coronary) heart disease. *Mod. Trends psychosom. Med., 3,* 208—329.

*23 Kimball, C.P. (1975) Psychological aspects of cardiovascular disease. In: *American Handbook of Psychiatry,* ed. S. Arieti, 2nd ed., vol. 4, pp. 608—17 New York: Basic Books.

24 Osler, W. (1897) *Lectures on Angina Pectoris and Allied States.* New York: Appleton.

25 Dunbar, F. (1943) *Psychosomatic Diagnosis.* New York: Hoeber.

26 Dunbar, F. (1946) *Emotions and Bodily Changes: A Survey of Literature on Psychosomatic Relationships 1910—1945,* 3rd ed. New York: Columbia University Press.

27 Alexander, F., French, T.M. & Pollock, G.H. (eds) (1968) *Psychosomatic Specificity: Vol. I: Experimental Study and Results.* Chicago and London: University of Chicago Press.

28 Graham, D.T., Lundy R.M. & Benjamin, L.D. (1962) Specific attitudes in initial interviews with patients having different 'psychosomatic diseases.' *Psychosom. Med., 24,* 257—66.

*29 Alexander, F. (1950) *Psychosomatic Medicine: Its Principles and Applications.* New York: Norton.

*30 Crisp, A.H. (1970) Some psychosomatic aspects of cancer. *Br. J. med. Psychol., 43,* 313—31.

*31 United States Department of Health, Education and Welfare (1973) *Psychological Aspects of Cancer: January 1970—March 1973.* Washington, D.C.

32 Schmale, A.H. jun. & Iker, H.P. (1976) The affect of hopelessness and the development of cancer: 1. identification of uterine cervical cancer in women with atypical cytology. *Psychosom. Med., 28,* 714—21.

Chapter 3: Meeting the patient

1 Revans, R. W. (1964) *Standards for Morale: Cause and Effect in Hospitals.* London: Oxford University Press for Nuffield Provincial Hospitals Trust.

2 White, A.G. (1953) The patient sits down: a clinical note. *Psychosom. Med., 15,* 256—7.

3 Byrne, P.S. & Long, B.E.L. (1976) *Doctors Talking to Patients: A Study of the Verbal Behaviour of General Practitioners Consulting in Their Surgeries.* London: HMSO.

*4 Fraser, C. (1976) An analysis of face-to-face communication. In: *Communication between Doctors and Patients,* ed. A.E. Bennett: London: Oxford University Press.

5   Joyce, C.R.B. (1964) What does the doctor let the patient tell him? *J. psychosom. Res., 8,* 343—52.

6   Balint, M. (1964) The doctor's therapeutic function. *Lancet, 1,* 1177—80.

7   Balint, M. (1964) *The Doctor, His Patient and the Illness,* 2nd ed. London: Pitman Medical.

*8   Ley, P. (1976) Towards better doctor-patient communications. In: *Communications between Doctors and Patients,* ed. A.E. Bennett. London: Oxford University Press.

*9   Blackwell, B. (1976) Treatment adherence. *Br. J. Psychiat., 129,* 513—31.

*10   British Medical Journal (1977) Keep on taking the tablets. *Br. med. J., 1,* 793.

11   Boyle, C.M. (1970) Differences between patients' and doctors' interpretation of some common medical terms. *Br. med. J., 2,* 286—98.

Chapter 4: Hospitals and their inhabitants

*1   Tuckett, D. (ed) (1976) *An Introduction to Medical Sociology.* London: Tavistock Publications

2   Price, J.I.W. (1977) The patient's morale. *Lancet, 1,* 533.

3   Raphael, W. (1977) *Patients and Their Hospitals.* London: King Edward's Hospital Fund for London.

4   Stockwell, F. (1972) *The Unpopular Patient.* London: Royal College of Nursing.

5   Goffman, E. (1961) *Asylums: Essays on the Social Situation of Mental Patients and Other Inmates.* New York: Doubleday— Anchor (Harmondsworth: Penguin, 1968).

6   Kesey, K. (1962) *One Flew Over the Cuckoo's Nest.* London: Methuen (Pan 1973).

*7   Cartwright, A. (1964) *Human Relations and Hospital Care.* London: Routledge and Kegan Paul.

8   Egebert, L.D., Battit, G.E., Welch, C.E. & Bartlett, M.K. (1964) Reduction of postoperative pain by encouragement and instruction of patients. *New Engl. J. Med., 270,* 825—7.

9   Revans, R.W. (1964) *Standards for Morale: Cause and Effect in Hospitals.* London: Oxford University Press.

10   Revans, R.W. (1964) The morale and effectiveness of general hospitals. In: *Problems and Progress in Medical Care,* ed. G. McLachlan. London: Oxford University Press.

11 Menzies, I.E.P. (1961) *The Functioning of Social Systems as a Defence against Anxiety: A Report on a Study of the Nursing Service of a General Hospital.* London: Tavistock Publications.

12 Crichton, A. & Crawford, M. (1963) *Disappointed Expectations? Report on a Survey of Professional and Technical Staff in the Hospital Service in Wales 1963.* Cardiff: Welsh Hospital Board, Welsh Staff Advisory Committee.

Chapter 5: Patients' responses to illness

1 Croog, S.H., Shapiro, D.S. & Levine, S. (1971) Denial among male heart patients : an empirical study. *Psychosom. Med., 33,* 385–97.

2 Titchener, J.L., Zwerling, L. & Gottschalk, L. (1956) Problem of delay in seeking surgical care. *J. Am. med. Ass.,160,* 1187–93.

3 Goldsen, R.K. (1963) Patient delay in seeking cancer diagnosis: behavioral aspects. *J. chron. Dis., 16,* 427–36.

4 Greer, S. (1974) Delay in the treatment of breast cancer. *Proc. R. Soc. Med., 67,* 470–3.

*5 Kutner, B., Makover, H.B. & Oppenheim, A. (1958) Delay in the diagnosis and treatment of cancer: A critical analysis of the literature. *J. chron. Dis., 7,* 95–120.

6 Kutner, B. & Gordon, G. (1961) Seeking care for cancer. *J. Hlth human Behav., 2,* 171–8.

7 Hackett, T.P., Cassem, N.H. & Raker, J.W. (1973) Patient delay in cancer. *New Engl. J. Med., 289,* 14–20.

8 Abrams, R.D. & Finesinger, J.E. (1953) Guilt reactions in patients with cancer. *Cancer, N.Y., 6,* 474–82.

9 Cobb, B., Clark, R.I., McGuire, C. & Howe, C.D. (1954) Patient-responsible delay of treatment in cancer: a social psychological study. *Cancer, N.Y., 7,* 920–6.

10 Henderson, J.G. (1966) Denial and repression as factors in the delay of patients with cancer presenting themselves to the physician. *Ann. N.Y. Acad. Sc., 125,* 856–64.

11 Henderson, J.G., Wittkower, E.D. & Loughed, M.N. (1958) A psychiatric investigation of the delay factor in patient to doctor presentation of cancer. *J. psychosom. Res., 3,* 27–41.

12 Robbins, G.F., Macdonald, M.C. & Pack, G.T. (1953) Delay in the diagnosis and treatment of physicians with cancer. *Cancer, N.Y., 6,* 624–6.

13 Alvarez, W.C. (1931) How early do physicians diagnose cancer of the stomach in themselves? *J. Am. med. Ass.*, 97, 77–83.

14 Byrd, B.F. (1951) Fatal pause in diagnosis of neoplastic disease in physician-patient. *J. Am. med. Ass.*, 147, 1219–20.

Chapter 6: Before the operation

1 Department of Health and Social Security (1976) *The Organisation of the In-Patient's Day.* London: HMSO.

2 Wood, P. (1956) *Disease of the Heart and Circulation*, 2nd ed. London: Eyre and Spottiswoode.

3 Hollingsworth, C., Hoffman, R., Scalzi, C. & Sokol, B. (1977) Patient progress rounds on a university cardiology service. *Am. J. Psychiat.*, 134, 42–4.

4 Querido, A. (1959) Forecast and follow up: an investigation into the clinical, social and mental factors determining the results of hospital treatment. *Br. J. prev. soc. Med.*, 13, 33–49.

5 McColl, I., Drinkwater, J.E., Hulme-Moir, I. & Donnan S.P.B. (1971) Prediction of success or failure of gastric surgery. *Br. J. Surg.*, 58, 768–71.

6 Pascal, G.R. & Thoroughman, J.C. (1967) Psychological studies of surgical intractability in duodenal ulcer patients. *Psychosomatics*, 8, 11–15.

7 Thoroughman, J.C., Pascal, G.R., Jenkins, W.O., Crutcher, J.C. & Peoples, L.C. (1964) Psychological factors predictive of surgical success in patients with intractable duodenal ulcer: a study of male veterans. *Psychosom. Med.*, 26, 618–24.

8 Kilpatrick, D.G., Miller, W.C., Allain, A.N., Huggins, M.B. & Lee, W.H. (1975) The use of psychological test data to predict open-heart surgery outcome: a prospective study. *Psychosom. Med.*, 37, 62–73.

9 Asher, R. (1951) Munchausen's syndrome. *Lancet*, 1, 339–41.

10 Blackwell, B. (1968) The Munchausen syndrome. *Br. J. Hosp. Med.*, 1, 98–102.

11 Enoch, M.D., Trethowan, W.H. & Barker, J.C. (1967) *Some Uncommon Psychiatric Syndromes.* Bristol: John Wright.

12 Barker, J.C. (1962) The syndrome of hospital addiction. *J. ment. Sci.*, 108, 167–82.

13 Menninger, K.A. (1934) Polysurgery and polysurgical addiction. *Psychoanal. Q.*, 3, 173–99.

14 Menninger, K.A. (1968) *Man Against Himself.* New York: Harcourt, Brace.

15 Ballinger, B.R. (1971) Minor self-injury. *Br. J. Psychiat., 118,* 535—8.

16 Kushner, A.W. (1967) Two cases of auto-castration due to religious delusions. *Br. J. med. Psychol., 40,* 293—8.

17 Gardner, A.J. (1967) Withdrawal fits in barbiturate addicts. *Lancet, 2,* 337—8.

18 Jefferson, J.W. (1975) A review of the cardiovascular effects and toxicity of tricyclic antidepressants. *Psychosom. Med., 37,* 160—79.

19 Tyrer, P. (1976) Towards rational therapy with monoamine oxidase inhibitors. *Br. J. Psychiat., 128,* 354—60.

20 Janis, I.I. (1958) *Psychological Stress: Psychoanalytic and Behavioral Studies of Surgical Patients.* New York: Wiley (London: Chapman and Hall).

21 Williams, J.G.L., Jones, J.R., Workhoven, M.N. & Williams, B. (1975) The psychological control of preoperative anxiety. *Psychophysiology, 12,* 50—4.

22 Abram, H.S. & Gill, B.F. (1961) Predictions of postoperative psychiatric complications. *New Engl. J. Med., 265,* 1123—8.

23 Schneider, R.A., Gray, J.S. & Culmer, C.U. (1950) Psychologic evaluation of surgical patients: a correlation between preoperative psychometric studies and recovery. *Wis. med. J., 49,* 285—90.

24 Titchener, J.L., Zwerling, I. & Gottschalk, L.A. (1957) Consequences of surgical illness and treatment: interaction of emotions, personality, and surgical illness, treatment and convalescence. *Archs Neurol. Psychiat., 77,* 623—34.

25 Cohen, F. & Lazarus, R.S. (1973) Active coping processes, coping dispositions, and recovery from surgery. *Psychosom. Med., 35,* 375—98.

26 Egbert, L.D., Battit, G.E., Welch, C.E. & Bartlett, M.K. (1964) Reduction of postoperative pain by encouragement and instruction of patients. *New Engl. J Med., 270,* 825—7.

Chapter 7: Postoperative care and intensive care

*1 Greene, R. (ed) (1971) *Sick Doctors.* London: Heinemann Medical.

2   Revans, R.W. (1964) *Standards for Morale: Cause and Effect in Hospitals.* London: Oxford.

3   Egbert, L.D., Battit, G.E., Welch, C.E. & Bartlett, M.K. (1964) Reduction of postoperative pain by encouragement and instruction of patients. *New Engl. J. Med., 270,* 825—7.

4   Lader, M.H. & Mathews, A.M. (1971) Electromyograph studies of tension. *J. psychosom. Res., 15,* 479—86.

5   Rahe, R.H. & Holmes, T. H. (1965) Social, psychologic and psychophysiologic aspects of inguinal hernia. *J. psychosom. Res., 8,* 487—91.

*6 Blanchard, E.B. & Young, L.D. (1974) Clinical applications of biofeedback training: a review of evidence. *Archs gen. Psychiat., 30,* 573—89.

7   Cobb, S. & McDermott, N.T. (1938) Postoperative psychosis. *Med. Clins N. Am., 22,* 569—76.

8   Knox, S.J. (1961) Severe psychiatric disturbance in the post-operative period — a five-year survey of Belfast hospitals. *J. ment. Sci., 107,* 1078—95.

9   Morse, R.M. & Litin, E.M. (1969) Postoperative delirium: a study of etiologic factors. *Am. J. Psychiat., 126,* 388—95.

10 Stengel, E., Zeitlyn, B.B. & Rayner, E.H. (1958) Postoperative psychoses. *J. ment. Sci., 104,* 389—402.

11 Titchener, J.L., Zwerling, I. & Gottschalk, L. (1956) Psychosis in surgical patients. *Surgery Gynec. Obstet., 102,* 59—65.

*12 Hazán, S.J. (1966) Psychiatric complications following cardiac surgery: (1) Review article. (2) A working hypothesis — the chemical approach. *J. thorac. cardiovasc. Surg., 51,* 308—25.

13 Kilpatrick, D.G., Miller, W.C., Allain, A.N., Huggins, M.B. & Lee, W.H. (1975) The use of psychological test data to predict open-heart surgery outcome: a prospective study. *Psychosom. Med., 37,* 62—73.

*14 Kornfeld, D.S., Heller, S.S., Frank, K.A. & Moskowitz, R. (1974) Personality and psychological factors in postcardiotomy delirium. *Archs gen. Psychiat., 31,* 249—53.

15 Morgan, D.H. (1971) Neuro-psychiatric problems of cardiac surgery. *J. psychosom. Res., 15,* 41—6.

16 Surman, O.S., Hacket, T.P., Silverberg, E.L. & Behrendt, D.M. (1974) Usefulness of psychiatric interview in patients undergoing cardiac surgery. *Archs gen. Psychiat., 30,* 830—5.

*17 Kornfeld, D.S. (1972) The hospital environment: its impact on the patient. *Adv. psychosom. Med., 8,* 252—70.

18 Leiber, L., Plumb, M.M., Gerstenzang, M.L. & Holland, J. (1976) The communication of affection between cancer patients and their spouses. *Psychosom. Med., 38*, 379—89.

19 Linn, L., Kahn, R.L., Coles, R., Cohen, J., Marshall, D. & Weinstein, E.A. (1953) Patterns of behavior disturbance following cataract extraction. *Am. J. Psychiat., 110*, 281—9.

20 Weisman, A.D. & Hackett, T.P. (1958) Psychosis after eye surgery: establishment of a specific doctor-patient relation in the prevention and treatment of 'black-patch' delirium. *New Engl. J. Med., 258*, 1284—9.

21 Bexton, W.H., Heron, W., & Scott, T.H. (1954) Effects of decreased variation in the sensory environment. *Can. J. Psychol., 8*, 70—6.

*22 Brownfield, C.A. (1965) *Isolation: Clinical and Experimental Approaches.* New York: Random House.

*23 Lilly, J.C. (1956) Mental effects of reduction of ordinary levels of physical stimuli on intact healthy persons. *Psychiat. Res. Rep., 5*, 1—28.

*24 Zubek, J.P. (ed.) (1969) *Sensory Deprivation: Fifteen Years of Research.* New York: Meredith Corporation.

*25 Baxter, S. (1974) Psychological problems of intensive care. *Br. J. Hosp. Med., 11*, 875—85.

26 Cassem, N.H. & Hackett, T.P. (1971) Psychiatric consultation in a coronary care unit. *Ann. intern. Med., 75*, 9—14.

27 Kornfeld, D.S. (1969) Psychiatric view of the intensive care unit. *Br. med. J., 1*, 108—10.

28 Kornfeld, D.S., Zimberg, S. & Malm, J.R. (1965) Psychiatric complications of open heart surgery. *New Engl. J. Med., 273*, 287—92.

29 Schroeder, H.G. (1971) Psycho-reactive problems of intensive therapy. *Anaesthesia, 26*, 28—35.

30 Hewitt, P. B. (1970) Subjective follow-up of patients from a surgical intensive therapy ward. *Br. med. J., 4*, 669—73.

31 Hackett, T.P., Cassem, N.H. & Wishnie, H.A. (1968) The coronary care unit: an appraisal of its pyschological hazards. *New Engl. J. Med., 279*, 1365—70.

32 Dominian, J. & Dobson, M. (1969) Study of patient's psychological attitudes to a coronary care unit. *Br. med. J., 4*, 795—98.

33 Klein, R.E., Kliner, V.A., Zipes, D.P, Troyer, W.G. & Wallace, G. (1968) Transfer from a coronary care unit: some adverse responses. *Archs intern. Med., 122*, 104—8.

34　Kaplan De-Nour, A. & Czaczkes, J.W. (1972) Personality factors in chronic haemodialysis patients causing noncompliance with medical regimen. *Psychosom. Med.*, *34*, 333—4.

35　Bernstein, N.R. (1976) *Emotional Care of the Facially Burned and Disfigured.* Boston: Little Brown.

36　Hay, D. & Oken, D. (1972) The psychological stresses of intensive care unit nursing. *Psychosom. Med.*, *34* 109—18.

Chapter 8: Pain

1　Illich, I. (1975) *Medical Nemesis: The Expropriation of Health.* London: Calder and Boyars.

2　Illich, I. (1977) *Limits to Medicine.* Harmondsworth: Penguin.

*3　Melzack, R. (1973) *The Puzzle of Pain.* Harmondsworth: Penguin.

*4　Beecher, H.K. (1959) *Measurement of Subjective Responses.* London: Oxford University Press.

5　Woodrow, K.M., Friedman, G.D., Sieglaub, A.B. & Collen, M.F. (1972) Pain tolerance: Differences according to age, sex and race. *Psychosom. Med.*, *34*, 548—56.

6　Zborowski, M. (1952) Cultural components in responses to pain. *J. soc. Issues*, *8*, 16—30.

*7　Merskey, H. (1976) The status of pain. *Mod. Trends psychosom. Med.*, *3*, 166—86.

8　Pilowsky, I. & Spence, N. D. (1976) Illness behaviour syndromes associated with intractable pain. *Pain*, *2*, 61—71.

9　Bradley, J.J. (1963) Severe localized pain associated with the depressive syndrome. *Br. J. Psychiat.*, *109*, 741—5.

10　Walters, A. (1961) Psychogenic regional pain alias hysterical pain. *Brain*, *84*, 1—18.

*11　Merskey, H. & Spear, F.G. (1967) *Pain: Psychological and Psychiatric Aspects.* London: Baillière, Tindall and Cassell.

12　Devine, R. and Merskey, H. (1965) The description of pain in psychiatric and general medical patients. *J. psychosom. Res.*, *9*, 311—6.

13　Hill, O.W. & Blendis, I. (1967) Physical and psychological evaluation of 'non-organic' abdominal pain. *Gut*, *8*, 221—9.

*14　Tecce, J.J. (1971) Contingent negative variation and individual differences. *Archs gen. Psychiat.*, *24*, 1—16.

15 Kiloh, L.G., McComas, A.J. & Osselton, J.W. (1972) *Clinical Electroencephalography*, 3rd ed. London: Butterworths.

16 Mushin, J. & Levy, R. (1974) Averaged evoked response in patients with psychogenic pain. *Psychol. Med. 4*, 19–27.

17 Bond, M.R. (1973) Personality studies in patients with pain secondary to organic disease. *J. psychosom. Res., 17*, 257–63.

18 Merskey, H. (1972) Personality traits of psychiatric patients with pain. *J. psychosom. Res., 16*, 163–6.

19 Woodforde, J.M. & Merskey, H. (1972) Personality traits of patients with chronic pain. *J. psychosom. Res., 16*, 167–72.

20 Engel, G.L. (1959) 'Psychogenic' pain and the pain-prone patient. *Am. J. Med., 26*, 899–918.

21 Davis, D.R. (1972) *Introduction to Psychopathology*. London: Oxford University Press.

Chapter 9: Aftermath of treatment

1 Parkes, C.M. (1975) Psycho-social transitions: comparison between reactions to loss of a limb and loss of a spouse. *Br. J. Psychiat., 127*, 204–10.

2 Parkes, C.M. & Napier, M.M. (1970) Psychiatric sequelae of amputation. *Br. J. Hosp. Med., 4*, 610–4.

3 Morgenstern, F.S. (1970) Chronic pain: a study of some general features which play a role in maintaining a state of chronic pain after amputation. *Mod. Trends psychosom. Med., 2*, 225–45.

4 Parkes, C.M. (1973) Factors determining the persistence of phantom pain in the amputee. *J. psychosom. Res., 17*, 97–108.

5 Ballinger, C.B. (1977) Psychiatric morbidity and the menopause: survey of a gynaecological out-patient clinic. *Br. J. Psychiat., 131*, 83–9.

6 Barker, M.G. (1968) Psychiatric illness after hysterectomy. *Br. med. J., 2*, 91–5.

7 Richards, D.H. (1973) Depression after hysterectomy. *Lancet, 2*, 430–3.

8 Richards, D.H. (1974) A post-hysterectomy syndrome. *Lancet, 2*, 983–5.

9 Asken, M.J. (1975) Psychoemotional aspects of mastectomy: a review of recent literature. *Am. J. Psychiat., 132*, 56–9.

10 Klein, R. (1971) A crisis to grow on. *Cancer, N.Y., 28*, 1660–5.

11 Maguire, G.P., Lee, E.G., Bevington, D.J., Küchemann, C.S., Crabtree, R.J. & Cornell, C.E. (1978) Psychiatric problems in the first year after mastectomy. *Br. med. J.*, *1*, 963—5.

12 Torrie, A. (1970) Like a bird with broken wings. *World Med.*, *5*, 36—47.

*13 Brand, P.C. & Van Keep, P.A. (eds.) (1978) *Breast Cancer: Psychosocial Aspects of Early Detection and Treatment.* Lancaster: MTP Press.

14 Dlin, B.M. (1973) Emotional aspects of colostomy and ileostomy. In: *Emotional Factors in Gastrointestinal Illness*, ed. A.E. Lindner. New York: Elsevier.

15 Briggs, M.K., Plant, J.A. & Devlin, H.B. (1977) Labelling the stigmatized: the career of the colostomist. *Ann. R. Coll. Surg.*, *59*, 247—50.

16 Druss, R.G., O'Connor, J.F., Prudden, J.F. & Stern, L.O. (1968) Psychologic response to colectomy: I. Ileostomy. *Archs gen. Psychiat.*, *18*, 53—9.

17 Druss, R.G., O'Connor, J.F. & Stern, L.O. (1969) Psychologic response to colectomy: II. Adjustment to a permanent colostomy. *Archs gen. Psychiat.*, *20*, 419—27.

18 Ritchie, J.K. (1971) Ileostomy and excisional surgery for chronic inflammatory disease of the colon: a survey of one hospital region. Part II, the health of ileostomatists. *Gut*, *12*, 536—40.

19 Sutherland, A.M., Orbach, C.E., Dyk, R.B. & Bard, M. (1952) The psychological impact of cancer and cancer surgery. I. Adaptation to the dry colostomy; preliminary report and summary of findings. *Cancer, N.Y.*, *5*, 857—72.

*20 Engel, G.L. (1973) Ulcerative colitis. In: *Emotional Factors in Gastrointestinal Illness*, ed. A.E. Lindner. New York: Elsevier.

*21 O'Connor, J.F. (1970) A comprehensive approach to the treatment of ulcerative colitis. *Mod. Trends psychosom. Med.*, *2*, 172—88.

*22 Whybrow, P.C. & Ferrell, R.B. (1973) Psychic factors and Crohn's disease: and overview. In: *Emotional Factors in Gastrointestinal Illness*, ed. A.E. Lindner. New York; Elsevier.

23 Goldberg, D. (1970) A psychiatric study of patients with diseases of the small intestine. *Gut*, *11*, 459—65.

24 Farley, D. & Smith, I. (1969) Phantom rectum after complete rectal excision. *Br. J. Surg.*, *55*, 40.

25 Devlin, H.B., Plant, J.A. & Griffin, M. (1971) Aftermath of surgery for anorectal cancer. *Br. med. J.*, *3*, 413—8.

26 Daly, D.W. (1968) The outcome of surgery for ulcerative colitis.
    Ann. R. Coll. Surg., 42, 38—57.

27 Druss, R.G., O'Connor, J.F. & Stern, I.O. (1972) Changes in body
    image following ileostomy. *Psychoanal. Q., 40*, 195—206.

28 Finkle, A.L. & Prian, D.V. (1966) Sexual potency in elderly men
    before and after prostatectomy. *J. Am. med. Ass., 196*, 139—43.

29 Gold, F.M. & Hotchkiss, R.S. (1969) Sexual potency following
    simple prostatectomy. *N. Y. St. J. Med., 69*, 2987—89.

30 Goligher, J.C. (1975) *Surgery of the Anus, Rectum and Colon*,
    3rd ed. London: Baillière, Tindall and Cassell.

31 Rankin, J.T. (1969) Urological complications of rectal surgery.
    Br. J. Urol., 41, 655—9.

32 Davis, L.P. & Jelenko, C. (1975) Sexual function after abdomino-
    perineal resection. *Sth med. J., 68*, 422—6.

33 Stahlgren, L.H. & Ferguson, L.K. (1958) Influence on sexual
    function of abdominoperineal resection for ulcerative colitis.
    New Engl. J. Med., 259, 873—5.

34 Harris, J.D. & Jepson, R.P. (1965) Aorto-iliac stenosis: a com-
    parison of two procedures. *Aust. N.Z. J. Surg., 34*, 211—4.

35 May, A.G., DeWeese, J.A. & Rob, C.G. (1969) Changes in sexual
    function following operation on the abdominal aorta. *Surgery, St
    Louis, 65*, 41.

36 Sabri, S. & Cotton, L.T. (1971) Sexual function following aort-
    iliac reconstruction. *Lancet, 2*, 1218—9.

37 Beischer, N.A. (1967) The anatomical and functional results of
    mediolateral episiotomy. *Med. J. Aust., 2*, 189—95.

*38 Amias, A.G. (1975) Sexual life after gynaecological operations I
    and II. *Br. med. J., 2*, 608—9, 680—1.

39 Abithol, M.M. & Davenport, J.H. (1974) Sexual dysfunction after
    therapy for cervical carcinoma. *Am. J. Obstet. Gynec., 119*,
    181—9.

40 Jeffacoate, T.N.A. (1959) Posterior colpoperineorrhaphy. *Am. J.
    Obstet. Gynec., 77*, 490—502.

41 Levy, N.B. (1974) Sexual adjustment to maintenance hemo-
    dialysis and renal transplantation: National survey by question-
    naire: Preliminary report. In: *Living or Dying: Adaptation to
    Hemodialysis*. Springfield, Ill.: Charles C Thomas.

42 Abram, H.S. (1974) The 'uncooperative' hemodialysis patient: a
    psychiatrist's viewpoint and a patient's commentary. In: *Living
    or Dying: Adaptation to Hemodialysis*, ed. N.B. Levy. Spring-
    field, Ill.: Charles C Thomas.

43 Levy, N.B. & Wynbrandt, G.D. (1975) The quality of life on maintenance haemodialysis. *Lancet, 1,* 1328—30.

44 Greenberg, H.R. (1965) Erectile impotence during the course of tofranil therapy. *Am. J. Psychiat., 121,* 1021.

Chapter 10: Beyond cure

1 Fitts, W.T. & Ravdin, I.S. (1953) What Philadelphia physicians tell patients with cancer. *J. Am. med. Ass., 153,* 901—4.

2 Oken, D. (1961) What to tell cancer patients: a study of medical attitudes. *J. Am. med. Ass., 175,* 1120—8.

3 Kelly, W.D. & Friesen, S.R. (1950) Do cancer patients want to be told? *Surgery, St Louis, 27,* 822—6.

4 Gilbertsen, V.A. & Wangensteen, O.H. (1962) Should the doctor tell the patient that the disease is cancer? *CA, 12,* 82—6.

5 Aitken-Swan, J. & Easson, E.C. (1959) Reactions of cancer patients on being told their diagnosis. *Br. med. J., 1,* 779—83.

6 Achté, K.A. & Vauhkonen, M.L. (1967) Cancer and the psyche. *Annls Med. intern. Fenn., 56,* Suppl. 48, 1—30.

7 Illich, I. (1975) *Medical Nemesis: The Expropriation of Health.* London: Calder and Boyars.

8 Illich, I. (1977) *Limits to Medicine.* Harmondsworth: Penguin.

9 Saunders, C. (1966/7) Management of terminal illness. *Hosp. Med., 1,* 225—8, 317—20, 433—6.

10 Saunders, C.M. (1976) The challenge of terminal care. In: *Scientific Foundations of Oncology,* ed. T. Symington & R.L. Carter. London: Heinemann Medical.

11 Cartwright, A., Hockey, L. & Anderson, J.L. (1973) *Life Before Death.* London: Routledge and Kegan Paul.

12 Caughill, R.E. (ed.) (1976) *The Dying Patient: A Supportive Approach.* Boston: Little, Brown.

13 Hinton, J. (1967) *Dying.* Harmondsworth: Penguin.

14 Hinton, J. (1976) Approaching death. *Mod. Trends psychosom. Med., 3,* 471—90.

15 Kübler-Ross, E. (1969) *On Death and Dying.* New York: Macmillan (London: Tavistock Publications, 1970).

16 Artiss, K.L. & Levine, A.S. (1973) Doctor—patient relation in severe illness: a seminar for oncology fellows. *New Engl. J. Med., 288,* 1210—14.

17 Smith, J.K. (1975) *Free Fall.* Valley Forge, Penn.: Judson (London: SPCK, 1977).

18 See also Pelgrin, M. (1961) *and a Time to Die.* London: Routledge and Kegan Paul. This is another personal account of dying.

Chapter 11: The honoured practitioner

1 *Royal Commission on Medical Education 1965—68* (1968) Cmnd. 3569. London: HMSO.

2 Adorno, T.W., Frenkel-Brunswik, E., Levinson, D.F. & Sanfird, R.N. (1950) *The Authoritarian Personality.* New York: Harper and Row.

3 Hudson, L. (1966) *Contrary Imaginations: A Psychological Study of the English Schoolboy.* London: Methuen (Harmondsworth: Penguin).

4 Hudson, L. (1968) *Frames of Mind: Ability, Perception and Self-Perception in the Arts and Sciences.* London: Methuen (Harmondsworth: Penguin).

5 Hooper, D. & Humphrey, M. (1968) Behavioural science for preclinical students. *Lancet, 2,* 1293—5.

6 Davis, D.R. (1970) Behavioural science in the preclinical curriculum. *Br. J. med. Educ., 4,* 194—7.

7 Nokes, P. (1967) *The Professional Task in Welfare Practice.* London: Routledge and Kegan Paul.

8 Ferris, P. (1965) *The Doctors,* London: Gollancz (Harmondsworth: Penguin).

9 Waitzkin, H. & Stoeckle, J.D. (1972) The communication of information about illness: clinical, sociological and methodological considerations. *Adv. psychosom. Med., 8,* 180—215.

10 Abram, H.S. (1974) The 'uncooperative' hemodialysis patient: a psychiatrist's viewpoint and a patient's commentary. In: *Living or Dying: Adaptation to Hemodialysis,* ed. N.B. Levy. Springfield, Ill.: Charles C. Thomas.

11 Balint, M. (1964) *The Doctor, His Patient and the Illness,* 2nd ed. London: Pitman Medical.

12 Guggenbuhl-Craig, A. (1971) *Power in the Helping Professions.* Zurich: Spring Publications.

13 Solzhenitsyn, A. (1971) *Cancer Ward.* London: The Bodley Head. (Harmondsworth: Penguin).

Chapter 12: Doctors in private

1   Osler, W. (1908) *Aequanimitas: with Other Addresses to Medical Students, Nurses and Practitioners of Medicine,* 2nd ed. London: H.K. Lewis.

2   Shapiro, E.T., Pinsker, H. & Shale, J.H. (1975) The mentally ill physician as practitioner. *J. Am. med. Ass., 232,* 725—7.

3   a'Brook, M.F., Hailstone, J.D. & McLauchlan, I.E.J. (1967) Psychiatric illness in the medical profession. *Br. J. Psychiat, 113,* 1013—23.

4   Duffy, J.C. & Litin, E.M. (1967) *The Emotional Health of Physicians.* Springfield, Ill.: Charles C Thomas.

5   Freeman, W. (1968) *The Psychiatrist: Personalities and Patterns.* New York: Grune and Stratton.

6   Murray, R.M. (1974) Psychiatric illness in doctors. *Lancet, 1,* 1211—2.

7   Pearson, M.M. & Strecker, E.A. (1960) Physicians as psychiatric patients: private practice experience. *Am. J. Psychiat., 116,* 915—9.

8   Small, I.F., Small, J.G., Assue, C.M. & Moore, D.F. (1969) The fate of the mentally ill physician. *Am. J. Psychiat., 125,* 1333—42.

9   Vaillant, G.E., Sobowale, N.C. & McArthur, C. (1972) Some psychologic vulnerabilities of physicians. *New Engl. J. Med., 287,* 372—5.

*10   Waring, E.W. (1974) Psychiatric illness in physicians: a review. *Comprehensive Psychiat., 15,* 519—30.

11   Modlin, H.C. & Montes, A. (1964) Narcotic addiction in physicians. *Am. J. Psychiat., 121,* 358—65.

12   Putnam, P.L. & Ellinwood, E.H. (1966) Narcotic addiction among physicians: a ten year follow up. *Am. J. Psychiat., 122,* 745—8.

13   Murray, R.M. (1977) The alcoholic doctor. *Br. J. Hosp. Med., 17,* 144—9.

14   *The Registrar General's Decennial Supplement. England and Wales 1961. Occupational Mortality* (1971). London: HMSO.

15   *The Registrar General's Decennial Supplement. England and Wales 1970—72. Occupational Mortality* (1978). London: HMSO.

16   Bissell, L. & Jones, R.W. (1976) The alcoholic physician: a survey. *Am. J. Psychiat., 133,* 1142—6.

17   Edwards, G. (1975) The alcoholic doctor: a case of neglect. *Lancet, 2,* 1297—8.

18 Bruce, D.L., Eide, K.A., Smith, N.J., Seltzer, F. & Dykes, M.H.M. (1974) A prospective survey of anesthesiologist mortality, 1967—1971. *Anesthesiology, 41,* 71—4.

19 Harrington, J.M. & Shannon, H.S. (1975) Mortality study of pathologists and medical laboratory technicians. *Br. med. J., 4,* 329—32.

20 Rose, K.D. & Rosow, I. (1973) Physicians who kill themselves. *Archs gen. Psychiat., 29,* 800—5.

21 von Brauchitsch, H. (1976) The physician's suicide revisited. *J. nervous ment. Dis., 162,* 40—5.

22 Epstein, L.C., Thomas, C.B., Shaffer, J.W. & Perlin, S.J. (1973) Clinical prediction of physician suicide based on medical student data. *J. nervous ment. Dis., 156,* 19—29.

23 McClinton, J.B. (1942) The doctor's own wife: his fourth investment. *Can. med. Ass. J., 47,* 472—6.

24 Miles, J.E., Krell, R. & Lin, T.Y. (1975) The doctor's wife: mental illness and marital pattern. *Intern. J. Psychiat. Med., 6,* 481—7.

25 Scarlett, E.P. (1965) The doctor's wife. *Archs intern. Med., 115,* 351—7.

26 Vincent, M.O. (1969) Doctor and Mrs. — their mental health. *Can. psychiat. Ass. J., 14,* 509—15.

27 Evans, J.L. (1965) Psychiatric illness in the physician's wife. *Am. J. Psychiat., 122,* 159—63.

28 Lewis, J.M. (1965) The doctor and his marriage. *Texas St. J. Med., 61,* 615—19.

29 Dalrymple-Champneys, D. (1959) Wives of some famous doctors. *Proc. R. Soc. Med., 52,* 937—46.

30 Osler, W. (1908) The student life. In: *Aequanimitas with Other Addresses to Medical Students, Nurses and Practitioners of Medicine,* 2nd ed. London: H.K. Lewis.

31 de Castillejo, I.C. (1973) *Knowing Woman: A Feminine Psychology.* London: Hodder and Stoughton.

Chapter 13: Fallibilities of doctors

1 Abercrombie, M.L.J. (1960) *The Anatomy of Judgement: An Investigation into the Processes of Perception and Reasoning.* London: Hutchinson.

2 Abercrombie, M.L.J. (1964) The observer and his errors. *J. psychosom. Res.*, *8*, 169—75.

3 Lusted, L.B. (1968) *Introduction to Medical Decision Making.* Springfield, Ill.: Charles C Thomas.

4 Birkelo, C.C., Chamberlain, W.F., Phelps, P.S., Schools, P.E., Zacks, D. & Yerushalmy, J. (1947) Tuberculosis case findings: a comparison of the effectiveness of various roentgenographic and photofluorographic methods. *J. Am. med. Ass.*, *133*, 359—66.

5 Yerushalmy, J., Garland, L.H. & Harkness, J.T. (1951) An evaluation of the role of serial chest roentgenograms in estimating the progress of disease in patients with pulmonary tuberculosis. *A. Rev. Tuberc.*, *64*, 225—48.

6 Graham, N.G., de Dombal, F.T. & Goligher, J.C. (1971) Reliability of physical signs in patients with severe attacks of ulcerative colitis. *Br. med. J.*, *2*, 746—8.

7 Wilkinson, R.T. (1969) Sleep deprivation and behaviour. In: *Progress in Clinical Psychology*, ed. B.F. Riess & L.A. Abt. New York: Grune and Stratton.

8 Wilkinson, R.T. (1966) Sleep and dreams. In: *New Horizons in Psychology*, ed. B.M. Foss. Harmondsworth: Penguin.

9 Friedman, R.C., Bigger, J.T. & Kornfeld, D.S. (1971) The intern and sleep loss. *New Engl. J. Med.*, *285*, 201—3.

10 Bennet, G. (1973) Medical and psychological problems in the 1972 singlehanded transatlantic yacht race. *Lancet*, *2*, 747—54.

11 Bennet, G. (1973) The tired sailor and the hazards of fatigue. *Yachting Monthly*, *133*, 1393—9; *Sail*, *4*, 69—76.

12 Davis, D.R. (1966) Railway signals passed at danger: the drivers, circumstances, and psychological processes. *Ergonomics*, *9*, 211—22.

13 Hersey, J. (1946) *Hiroshima.* Harmondsworth: Penguin.

14 Wallace, A.F.C. (1956) *Tornado in Worcester: An Exploratory Study in Individual and Community Behavior in an Extreme Situation.* Disaster Study No. 3. Washington, D.C.: National Academy of Sciences, National Research Council.

15 Popper, K.R. (1972) *Conjectures and Refutations: The Growth of Scientific Knowledge*, 4th ed. London: Routledge and Kegan Paul.

*16 Comfort, A. (1967) *The Anxiety Makers.* London: Nelson (Panther, 1968).

*17 Hare, F.H. (1962) Masturbational insanity: the history of an idea. *J. ment. Sci.*, *108*, 1—25.

18 Hillman, J. (1975) *Loose Ends: Primary Papers in Archetypal Psychology.* Zurich: Spring Publications.

19 *Cannabis: Report by the Advisory Committee on Drug Dependence* (1968). London: HMSO.

20 Mitchell, S.W. (1896) Remarks on the effects of Anhalonium Lewinii (the mescal button). *Br. med. J.,* 2, 1625–9.

21 Ellis, H. (1897) Mescal: a new artifical paradise. *Ann. Rep. Smithsonian Institution.*

22 Campbell, A.M.G., Evans, M., Thomson, J.L.G. & Williams, M.J. (1971) Cerebral atrophy in young cannabis smokers. *Lancet,* 2, 1219–24.

*23 Blandy, J.P. (1968) Circumcision. *Hosp. Med.,* 2, 551–3.

*24 Gairdner, D. (1949) The fate of the foreskin: a study in circumcision. *Br. med. J.,* 2, 1433–7.

25 Ozturk, O.M. (1973) Ritual circumcision and castration anxiety. *Psychiatry,* 36, 49–60.

Chapter 14: The wounded physician

1 Neumann, E. (1955) *The Great Mother: An Analysis of the Archetype.* London: Routledge and Kegan Paul.

2 Laing, R.D. & Esterson, A. (1964) *Sanity, Madness, and the Family: Families of Schizophrenics.* London: Methuen (Harmondsworth: Penguin).

*3 Castiglioni, A. (1947) *A History of Medicine.* New York: A. Knopf.

4 Kerenyi, C. (1959) *Asklepios: Archetypal Image of the Physician's Existence.* New York: Pantheon.

5 Guggenbuhl-Craig, A. (1971) *Power in the Helping Professions.* Zurich: Spring Publications.

6 Bergin, A.E. & Garfield, S.L. (1971) *Handbook of Psychotherapy and Behavior Change.* New York: John Wiley.

7 Eliade, M. (1964) *Shamanism: Archaic Techniques of Ecstasy.* London: Routledge and Kegan Paul.

8 Lewis, I.M. (1971) *Ecstatic Religion: an Anthropological Study of Spirit Possession and Shamanism.* Harmondsworth: Penguin.

9 I Peter 2.24.

Name Index

209

Name Index

Subject Index

213